dr foster

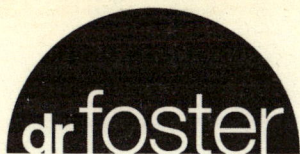

Your Guide to Better Health

DR FOSTER
FERTILITY
GUIDE

1 3 5 7 9 10 8 6 4 2

Copyright © 2002 by Dr Foster Ltd

First published 2002 by Vermilion,
an imprint of Ebury Press, Random House,
20 Vauxhall Bridge Road, London SW1V 2SA
www.randomhouse.co.uk
Random House Australia (Pty) Limited
20 Alfred Street, Milsons Point, Sydney,
New South Wales 2061, Australia
Random House New Zealand Limited
18 Poland Road, Glenfield, Auckland 10, New Zealand
Random House South Africa (Pty) Limited
Endulini, 5a Jubilee Road, Parktown 2193, South Africa

The Random House Group Limited Reg. No. 954009

Papers used by Vermilion are natural, recyclable products made from wood grown in sustainable forests.

Printed and bound in Great Britain by
Bookmarque Ltd, Croydon, Surrey

A CIP catalogue record for this book is available
from the British Library
ISBN 0091883814

How can I order more Dr Foster titles?
To order copies of any of these books direct from the publisher, call The Book Service credit card hotline on 01206 255800. Dr Foster guides are also available from all good booksellers.

drfoster

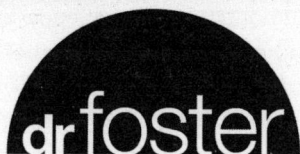

Your Guide to Better Health

DR FOSTER
FERTILITY
GUIDE

Researched and Compiled
by Dr Foster
Text by Patsy Westcott

Vermilion
LONDON

Who is Dr Foster?

Dr Foster provides authoritative information on health services of all kinds in the UK. Our aim is to empower patients with information to help them access the best possible care. We are supervised by a totally independent ethics committee comprising leading figures from the healthcare profession that has independent legal powers to ensure that guides meet the highest standards.

The ethics committee currently comprises the following membership:

Dr Jack Tinker, dean of the Royal Society of Medicine and chair of the committee
Sir Donald Irvine, past president, General Medical Council
Dr Michael Dixon, chair, NHS Alliance
Peter Griffiths, chief executive, Health Quality Service
Dianne Hayter, member of the board of the National Patient Safety Agency and the National Consumer Council
Professor Alan Maynard, director, Health Policy Unit, York University and chair, York Health Services NHS Trust
Wilma MacPherson, visiting professor at King's College London and a consultant in Health Services
Bridget Gill, chair of the Northern and Yorkshire Regional Council of the Institute of Healthcare Management
Trevor Campbell Davis, chief executive, Whittington Hospital
Douglas Webb, operations and development director, Friends of the Elderly

Vanessa Bourne, chair, Patients Association
Dr Philip Davies, medical director, Pontypridd and Rhondda NHS Trust
Professor Nairn Wilson, president of the General Dental Council

---

Dr Foster Help at Hand Service

Dr Foster information is regularly updated. To search the database go to **www.drfoster.co.uk** or call the **Help at Hand Service** line on **0906 190 0212**

Calls cost £1.50 per minute; costs from mobile phones and some other networks may be more. Callers must be aged 18 or over. Lines are open Mon to Fri from 8.30am – 8pm, Sat 8.30am – 6pm.

We can help with information on hospital and maternity services, infertility treatment centres and individual hospital doctors.

Dr Foster Ltd.
Sir John Lyon House
5 High Timber Street
London EC4V 3NX

Contents

Acknowledgements

Dr Foster would like to thank the following people for their time and help in compiling the information in this book (they are not, however, in any way responsible for anything included or omitted).

Clare Brown is Executive Director of CHILD, the National Infertility Support Network, joining in 1980 after being diagnosed as infertile. She had 2 attempts at tubal surgery and 4 attempts at IVF, going on to adopt her two children James and Holly in 1986. She holds several other infertility committee posts including the Presidency of the International Federation of Infertility Patient Associations, and has had several papers published in medical journals.

Dr Carole Gilling-Smith is a Consultant Gynaecologist and Director of the ACU at the Chelsea & Westminster Hospital. She trained at Trinity College, Cambridge, and Addenbrookes Hospital Medical School, graduating in 1984. She is UK co-ordinator for the European network of centres managing infertile couples with hepatitis or HIV. She has published review articles and papers on PCOS, early pregnancy bleeding, pelvic pain and HIV and infertility.

Gunhild Lenz-Mulligan underwent IVF treatment for over a year without success and has since adopted two children. Formerly an active member of ISSUE, she is now involved in Adoption UK.

Olivia Montuschi is a mother of two teenagers conceived through donor insemination and co-founder of the Donor Conception Network, a national self-help organisation that supports parents in being open with their children about their origins. She has written extensively in this field for parents and professionals and regularly broadcasts in the media on donor conception issues.

Elizabeth Rowe is a freelance editor and writer. She lives in London where she has been undergoing fertility treatment for four years.

Helene Torr is a founder of ACeBabes, a Regional Organiser for CHILD and runs the East Midlands Infertility Group. She has a four-year old son and two-year old-twins conceived through IVF.

Patsy Westcott is a writer and journalist. She regularly contributes to the national press, has written over 20 books on health and contributed to several health encyclopaedias and part-works.

Foreword by Clare Brown

To be told that you may not be able to have a family can be a devastating shock. Going through the investigations and treatment is often referred to as an emotional rollercoaster, and then there is the physical impact of infertility treatment. It is, therefore, important that couples empower themselves with factually correct and practical information. The *Doctor Foster Fertility Guide* does precisely that. It not only provides the medical information that patients need, but also vital and practical information on how to access emotional support such as counselling and support networks, which is so often lacking.

It also covers the important aspect of NHS funding (or current lack of it) and the various financial options available. So often assumptions are made that treatment will either be paid for by the NHS, or the opposite – that it must only be available privately. Such is the chaotic system we have at the moment. Those experiencing fertility problems need guidance and information of the sort contained in this book.

CHILD receives more and more requests for information on complementary therapies and the role they can play in the management of infertility. Few books provide this, so it is particularly gratifying to see such comprehensive coverage which will be so useful to many patients.

This book is a fantastic guide through the maze of infertility treatment right from the moment that a problem is suspected, through to the realisation that the family that is so desperately wanted may not be possible to achieve. Practical information and coping mechanisms are here throughout.

I recommend that all concerned should read, mark, learn and inwardly digest the information and advice in this excellent book.

Understanding Fertility Treatment

Introduction by Elizabeth Rowe

When you feel you're ready for parenthood but children just don't seem to be materialising, it may suddenly feel as though there are babies everywhere. Every woman you pass in the street is either pregnant or pushing a buggy and every shop is packed with cute Babygros and tiny leather shoes. Added to this, sensationalist headlines such as 'Miracle New Treatment Brings Hope to Childless Couples' or 'Good Nutrition Doubles Pregnancy Rate' can't fail to grab your attention.

If you have picked up this book, then it's likely that this is the situation you currently find yourself in. Perhaps getting pregnant is taking longer than you feel it should and you suspect that there's something wrong. You may have decided that you need to seek help and are not quite sure what to do next. Or maybe you've already embarked on a course of fertility treatment and would like to find out more about what's ahead of you. Either way, the phrase 'emotional roller coaster' is one that you're likely to hear repeated at fairly frequent intervals over the next few months or years.

The *Dr Foster Fertility Guide* has been specifically designed to provide you with all the information you need at such a bewildering time. It will help you make decisions about what treatment is best for you, where to go to be treated and how to deal with all the inevitable practical and emotional upheavals.

Unfortunately, more and more people are finding themselves in the position of having to explore fertility treatment. Currently, one in six couples are reported to have problems conceiving. Some of these couples will have their problem easily diagnosed and solved but that still leaves many having to face the long and torturous journey of fertility treatment. Sadly, only 20 per cent of those who go through assisted conception treatment will actually succeed in taking a baby home with them.

Why are so many couples finding it so hard to conceive naturally? Is infertility actually on the increase, or is it just the case that today's child-bearing generation is more likely to seek help in the hope that something can be done? Sperm counts are said to be declining year on year, possibly due to environmental factors such as pollutants in water and the use of agricultural pesticides and fertilisers. However, the most significant factor for any apparent rise in infertility is probably age. In 1974, the average age at which a woman gave birth was 26. In 2002, this has increased to 29. Nowadays, most women have been working for a number of years by the time they are ready to start a family. With some studies suggesting that female fertility starts to decline sharply at the age of 30, age is undoubtedly one of the most important factors to be taken into consideration when seeking fertility treatment.

However, even if you are slightly older than you'd like to be, there is still much that can be done. Since the birth of Louise Brown, the world's first test-tube baby, in 1978, there have been huge advances in reproductive medicine and the technology of conception. Patrick Steptoe and Robert Edwards, the test-tube baby makers, were the pioneers of IVF or in vitro fertilisation, a technique that is now used to treat approximately 20,000 people in the UK every year. In 1984, the first baby conceived as the result of egg donation (using eggs donated by one woman to another) was born in Australia. New techniques are being developed all the time and in the last decade it became possible to inject a single sperm directly into an egg, and even to transplant ovarian tissue. In June 2002 the first 'frozen egg' baby was born in the Midlands. Looking to the future, there is likely to be much more work on cloning and on pre-implantation genetic diagnosis (screening embryos for possible genetic disorders before they are implanted in the womb).

The pace of change has been incredibly rapid, so rapid that in 1984 a Committee of Enquiry, chaired by Mary Warnock, was set up to look into the moral and ethical issues being raised. There was concern about the danger of allowing such radical technology to proceed unchecked, especially when it could potentially affect so many people. There were worries that treatment was unsafe and that clinics were not being properly checked. Although the 1990 Human Fertilisation and Embryology Act went a long way towards regulating the system and thus calming fears, fertility treatment is still surrounded by controversy. One of the Warnock Committee Report's main recommendations was that a statutory body should be established and in 1991 the Human Fertilisation and Embryology Authority (HFEA) was founded, its express purpose being to keep an eye on the ethical, legal, social and medical ramifications of fertility treatment.

It is more than likely that you will come into contact with the HFEA in the course of your treatment. An independent organisation funded partly by clinics and partly by the government, the HFEA is responsible for inspecting existing centres for treatment and research and licensing new ones. It also keeps a formal register of (and receives a fee from) all those undergoing treatment and holds details of those who have donated eggs or sperm. You may want to contact the HFEA for information and advice. A reassuring presence, it acts as a symbol of the progress that has been made since the days when not getting pregnant meant either adoption or childlessness.

Despite the speed with which things have changed in the past few decades, much research still remains to be done. Twenty per cent of couples are told that their infertility is 'unexplained'. Some of these couples will endure a long and frustrating series of treatments without ever really knowing what is wrong with them. And it is not only the causes of infertility that require further research. Professor Robert Winston of the Hammersmith Hospital highlights implantation as a process that is still imperfectly understood. At least 40 per cent (and the figure may possibly be as high as 80 per cent) of all human embryos fail to implant, but the reasons why are still unclear. Similarly, the rate of miscarriage remains higher in pregnancies achieved with assisted conception than in natural pregnancies, with as many as 15 per cent of all IVF pregnancies miscarrying.

There is some positive news, however. The UK is definitely a good place to seek treatment. Generally regarded as being at the forefront of the research field, it hosts a number of teaching hospitals as well as a fair scattering of those regarded as the big names in fertility treatment. The UK's good reputation attracts hundreds of 'reproductive tourists' to this country every year. They may also be trying to circumvent the restrictions imposed in their own countries. For example, in Norway IVF is limited to married couples and patients under the age of 38 and in Sweden the use of donor eggs or sperm in IVF is banned.

However, the traffic goes both ways: every year dozens of Britons seek treatment abroad, wishing to escape the UK's long waiting lists for treatments such as egg donation, and to avoid the limits on embryo replacement (which currently stands at two in the UK, or three in exceptional circumstances). Many of them head for Spain where clinics provide interpreters and help with finding accommodation. For these people, the stress of the travelling and of undergoing a medical procedure in a foreign country is outweighed by the lure of the 60 per cent success rate claimed for egg donation. Yet such success does not come cheap.

Unfortunately there is generally a hefty price tag attached to fertility treatment, and this applies in the UK as well as overseas. Money is an unavoidable issue in this area of medicine and you will rapidly realise that infertility is a commercial business involving large fees and even larger salaries. In 1996 it was reported that 90 per cent of IVF treatment was privately funded. Given that a single course of IVF can cost as much as £4,000 (including the cost of the drugs), this means that it is simply beyond the reach of large numbers of people. The only options for these couples or individuals may be NHS-funded treatment.

Another example of the so-called 'postcode lottery', NHS-funded treatment is hard to come by. It is not unusual to find that a couple in one postal district has been offered a free cycle of IVF, while another living just 50 miles away has been told that the NHS cannot even cover the cost of the drugs. Such decisions are now made not by Health Authorities but by the local Primary Care Trusts (PCTs) who have taken over responsibilty for planning and developing local health services. Different PCTs impose different criteria on patients seeking funding so that, for example, upper age limits for women seem to vary between 34 and 43.

Your best bet is to discuss the funding issue with your GP as early as possible. Find out what treatment, if any, is available to you on the NHS and also enquire about self-funding (see p.162). Another avenue worth exploring is egg sharing, whereby in return for sharing your eggs with another woman, your own IVF treatment will be provided at reduced cost or possibly free of charge. The more information you can gather, the higher your chances of getting a fair deal.

The 'eccentrically variable' nature of the system is currently the target of NIAC (the National Infertility Awareness Campaign), who are campaigning for infertility treatment to be made available across the country in an equitable manner so that everyone has access to it. The provision and cost of treatment has long been the cause of debate, with some arguing that IVF patients should be low priority. It is said that the needs of people with fertility problems are social rather than medical and that, its budgets already overstretched, the NHS needs to concentrate on other, more pressing problems.

NIAC is supported in its campaign by CHILD, the National Infertility Support Network, and by ISSUE, the National Fertility Association. Both these organisations were set up to supply unbiased information, advice and support to all those experiencing difficulties with conception. They provide helplines run by experienced volunteers and produce useful and informative literature that helps to highlight the issues surrounding infertility and to raise public awareness. The support they offer may well be invaluable to you during what can be a very lonely and isolating period.

Fertility treatment is undoubtedly tough. You can find yourself on a high one day after a good scan and then in the depths of despair a few days later when your hormone levels have plummeted without warning. Managing your expectations is very difficult when time keeps ticking away and every attempt costs you thousands more pounds. Buoyed up with hope, perhaps after many years of fruitless attempts, anyone undergoing treatment is incredibly vulnerable emotionally. Anything to do with babies and children is highly charged, especially when you feel as though this really might represent your last chance to have your own happy, healthy infant. One very useful resource will be the counselling services that the HFEA Act of 1990 decreed every clinic should make available free of charge (see p.150).

Learning to view your treatment dispassionately is not easy (especially when you find yourself spending long periods of time in clinics whose walls are crammed with photos of cute babies) but it is valuable. It will enable you to take a practical approach to your treatment and to make the many necessary decisions sensibly and calmly. I became aware, within a year or so of setting out myself, that I was simply waiting for the system to sweep me along, for the doctors to give me instructions that I could follow. Such submission is natural when every doctor's appointment makes you feel tearful and mastering your emotions is as much as you can handle. But, as Anna Furse says in *The Infertility Companion: A User's Guide to Tests, Technology and Therapies* (Thorsons, £9.99), 'being victims makes us bad patients'. You will emerge a stronger person, whether you have become a parent or not, if you feel you have been able to get the best out of the system.

Taking charge of your own fertility treatment does not mean questioning everything you are told by your doctors. It just means having enough knowledge of your own to cope with the technical jargon and understand exactly what you are being told. During the course of four years of fertility treatment I have often felt as though I were just another numbered patient zipping past on a conveyor belt. Although I have never doubted my doctors' medical skills, I have sometimes felt excluded from my own treatment by their inability to communicate. Doctors themselves are often aware of this, as confirmed by Dr Ruth Curson, who wrote in her Foreword to *The Infertility Companion* (Thorsons, £9.99), 'As doctors, we forget that what seems logical and right to us may seem incomprehensible and frightening to others.' This point was brought home to me most forcefully when a specialist at a new clinic I'd just signed up to casually mentioned that it was obvious from the scans that my ovaries had shrunk. He was amazed when I burst into tears and was initially unable to comprehend why I found this concept so upsetting. Fertility treatment is a bewildering maze and a little information can make it much simpler to navigate your way through.

Taking control also means making practical arrangements for your treatment that are going to suit you. If you decide to opt for private treatment, one of the most important decisions you will probably have to take is which clinic to attend. The HFEA advises you to base that choice not on the success rates advertised by the clinic but on more everyday factors such as how close it is to your home, how much each individual cycle costs, what the atmosphere is like and what kind of treatments are on offer. You will only be adding to the stress of your treatment if you put your name down at a place that is many miles away and impossible to reach through rush-hour traffic.

No one is ever going to pretend that fertility treatment is fun. It is both expensive and intrusive, often inconvenient and sometimes uncomfortable. However, it is for many people a necessary evil, something they have to go through if they are to have any chance of fulfilling their desire for children. This book aims to make that journey slightly easier and less painful, to reassure you that you are far from alone and that support is on hand when needed and, hopefully, give you the confidence to make your ride on the fertility roller coaster as smooth as possible.

How to use this guide

This guide is unique. It has been specifically designed to explain what fertility treatment is and how to choose where to have it. Section one takes a fully comprehensive look at the different kinds of fertility treatment available in the UK and the issues you need to be aware of while seeking it. For instance, if your GP advises you to keep trying to conceive before referral to a specialist, should you follow their advice or try to get yourself on a waiting list via another GP? If NHS funding is not available in your area, which NHS clinics will allow you to 'self-fund', a way of paying less than you would have to for private treatment. If you are choosing a private clinic, how much attention should you pay to the live birth rate figures published in the glossy brochure? Is there any way of getting your fertility drugs more cheaply? And, if you are advised to go for assisted conception, should you explore alternatives before going down that route?

In section two we tell you about nearly every clinic in the country licensed by the HFEA. For each clinic we list the latest information on the treatments and services they provide. We tell you how much they cost, whether you will be eligible for treatment and how long you will have to wait for it. Also in this section we include information on individual fertility specialists, and explain what kind of NHS funding is available in your area.

The guide aims to be as comprehensive as possible. However, for ease of editorial style, it assumes that the couple seeking fertility treatment are heterosexual and refers to the primary reader as female and to their partner as male. This is in no way intended to alienate the growing number of single women and lesbians who seek fertility treatment every year.

Whatever your fertility problems and wherever you live, the Dr Foster Fertility Guide tells you everything you need to know to make the most informed choices possible.

Understanding fertility

To understand why some couples have problems conceiving, it helps to appreciate what needs to happen for conception to occur. Equally, knowing what the various hormones are and how they interact with each other can help you understand the origins and the treatment of many cases of infertility.

To maximise the chances of conception, a sperm needs to meet an egg (or ovum) around the time of ovulation (the release of an egg from the ovaries). An egg can be fertilised for just 12 to 24 hours after ovulation, while on average, sperm have fertilising capacity for 12 to 48 hours once ejaculated into the vagina. This leaves a window of just three days – no more than 48 hours before ovulation and no more than 24 hours after – during which fertilisation can occur. This is your body's way of enhancing the chances of pregnancy. It means that it is still possible to get pregnant whether you have sex before or after ovulation.

When does ovulation happen?

Normally ovulation occurs 14 days before a period. So, if you have an average menstrual cycle of 28 days, it will take place on or around day 14. If you have a cycle of 35 days, it will take place round about day 21, and if you have a cycle of 21 days, it will take place on approximately day seven.

What part do hormones play in fertility?

Hormones are chemical messengers, released by the glands of the endocrine or hormonal system, that act on organs far from their site of origin. Among other things, they control the release of eggs in women and sperm in men.

The body's glands all work together to make sure that the body stays in a constant state of balance. This is made possible by a series of 'feedback loops' that slow or stop the activity of a gland once enough of its hormone has been produced, and turn it on again when more hormone is needed, rather like a central heating thermostat.

The menstrual cycle and the production of sperm are both under the control of a three-way feedback loop which operates between three key organs:

- **the hypothalamus**, the part of the brain that orchestrates the body's hormone production
- **the pituitary**, the body's master gland that stimulates the action of other glands
- **the gonads** – these are the ovaries in women and the testes in men

How do these work together?

The hypothalamus is a cherry-sized region of the brain with nerve connections to most other parts of the nervous system. It is connected to the pituitary gland by a short stalk of nerve fibres. The hypothalamus secretes a number of chemicals called hormone-releasing factors, which control the secretion of hormones from the pituitary. One of these is gonadotrophin-releasing hormone, or GnRH, which stimulates the pituitary to produce two other key hormones for fertility: follicle-stimulating hormone (FSH) and luteinising hormone (LH).

The pituitary is a pea-sized gland at the base of the brain. It is often referred to as the body's master gland because it regulates and controls the activities of all the other endocrine glands. Among the many hormones the pituitary secretes are two key hormones for fertility in both the female and the male. These are:

- follicle-stimulating hormone, or FSH, which stimulates the maturation of follicles (or egg sacs) in the ovaries in women and stimulates the manufacture of sperm in men.
- luteinising hormone, or LH, which stimulates the release of eggs through the ovary wall in women and supports the production of the sex hormone testosterone and the production of sperm in men.

FSH and LH are known as gonadotrophins. They form the basis of the fertility drugs that are widely used to treat female and, less often, male infertility.

The ovaries are reproductive organs, that store and produce eggs. They are also glands, and produce the hormones oestrogen and progesterone.

The testes are reproductive organs, that produce sperm. They are also glands that produce testosterone, a sex hormone that is responsible for the sex drive and male sexual characteristics such as hair growth, muscles and a deep voice.

What are follicles and what do they do?

A follicle is the fluid-filled sac in the ovary that develops in each menstrual cycle and produces a mature egg capable of being fertilised. Each follicle contains an immature egg that can potentially develop in the future. At birth, all the follicles you will ever produce are present in your ovaries. Most of these will lie dormant but some will develop and the eggs inside them start to ripen. In a natural menstrual cycle, one follicle will become dominant and the egg inside it will ripen to maturity to be released at ovulation. Many others die through a process of natural wastage, with the result that as time goes on the number of dormant follicles in the ovaries falls until the menopause when they run out altogether.

What part do hormones play in the female fertility cycle?

On the first day of the menstrual cycle, falling levels of oestrogen and progesterone trigger the pituitary to produce FSH. FSH travels in the bloodstream to the ovaries where it stimulates about 20 follicles (or egg sacs) to grow. It also triggers the secretion of oestrogen by the ovaries.

In turn, rising levels of oestrogen in the blood cause a lowering of FSH, precisely measured to allow one follicle and its egg to ripen. At the same time oestrogen causes the womb lining (endometrium) to thicken in preparation for receiving a fertilised egg.

As oestrogen levels begin to peak – around mid-cycle – they trigger a sudden surge of luteinising hormone, or LH, from the pituitary gland. This stimulates the ripened egg to burst from its follicle (ovulation) into the fallopian tube about 36 to 42 hours later.

After ovulation, LH stimulates the development of the corpus luteum (Latin for yellow body) in the empty follicle. In order to help establish a pregnancy, the corpus luteum makes and releases its own hormone, progesterone, which increases the blood supply to the endometrium ready for an embryo to implant.

The egg can be fertilised for 24 hours after ovulation. If it is not fertilised – or if it is fertilised but fails to implant in the uterus – the corpus luteum shrinks, the egg disintegrates, and progesterone levels plummet. This in turn causes the blood vessels in the endometrium to break up and the uterus fills with blood and tissue. The uterine walls contract to expel this in the form of a menstrual period. Progesterone and oestrogen levels decline, halting the blockade of FSH and LH and the whole cycle starts anew.

What part do hormones play in male fertility?

The production of sperm and of the male sex hormone, testosterone, is regulated by the very same feedback loop between the hypothalamus, the pituitary and the gonads (in men, the testes) as female fertility. However, whereas women are born with a full complement of eggs, sperm is produced all the time. In fact, a healthy adult male makes about 400 million sperm each and every day. As a result, sperm can be vulnerable to infections and lifestyle factors such as smoking, drinking and recreational drugs, exposure to industrial chemicals and illness.

How are sperm made?

The hypothalamus releases gonadotrophin-releasing hormone (GnRH) which acts on the pituitary. The pituitary responds by releasing FSH and LH into the bloodstream. FSH acts on cells in a part of the testes called the seminiferous tubules or Sertoli's cells, causing them to produce sperm. LH acts on other cells (known as the interstitial cells), causing them to produce testosterone (and a small amount of oestrogen). This is why in men, LH is sometimes known as interstitial cell-stimulating hormone, or ICSH. Within the testes testosterone acts as the final trigger for sperm to be made.

Testosterone blocks the release of GnRH in the hypothalamus and may also act directly on the pituitary to inhibit gonadotrophin release. When the sperm count is high, another hormone – inhibin – increases, blocking the release of FSH by the pituitary and of GnRH by the hypothalamus. When sperm count falls below 20 million per millilitre, inhibin secretion declines, allowing sperm formation or spermatogenesis to begin again. The whole process takes 64 to 72 days.

The sperm cells produced in the seminiferous tubules are unable to swim and cannot fertilise an egg. They mature as they are forced by the pressure of testicular fluid through the tubular system of the testes and into the epididymis. This is a single coiled tube around 40 ft (12 m) long that leads to the penis. The contractions of the epididymis modify the sperm, causing them to become able to move (motile) and capable of fertilisation. If the epididymis is damaged, sperm may not be able to develop normally and so be incapable of fertilisation. If blocked, all sperm production from that testis is useless. The epididymis is joined by another tube (the vas deferens) which contracts during male orgasm to force sperm out through the penis.

How does fertilisation occur?

In order for fertilisation to occur, sperm must reach the egg. This is not always quite as simple as it sounds. At ejaculation, the vas deferens and the urethra (the tube that carries both urine and sperm through the penis to the outside of the body) contract powerfully, forcing sperm and seminal fluid out in spurts. Up to 300 million sperm are ejaculated into the vagina. However, only a few hundred will ever penetrate the cervical mucus and swim into the uterus. This seemingly enormous loss is a safeguard to ensure that only the strongest, fittest sperm have the chance to fertilise the egg. Millions of sperm leak from the vagina straightaway. Of the remainder, millions more are destroyed by the acidic secretions of the vagina, which is naturally hostile to sperm. Yet more millions will fail at the cervix, which has to be made fluid and slippery by the hormone oestrogen, in order to aid the sperm's journey. Those that do make it through the uterus are dispersed by contractions throughout the uterine cavity, where thousands more are destroyed by the white blood cells of the immune system. Just a few thousand – and sometimes fewer – make it into the fallopian tubes where the egg is moving down towards the uterus. By the time they reach the egg at the outer end of the fallopian tube where fertilisation normally occurs, just 500 to 1000 remain.

As if this isn't complicated enough, sperm also have another difficulty to overcome. Sperm freshly ejaculated into the vagina are incapable of penetrating an egg. In order to do so, eggs have to undergo a process called capacitation in which their membranes become fragile.

Enzymes within the 'sperm cap' are released, which break down the outer 'shell' or zona pellucida of the egg, clearing a path for the single successful sperm which will fuse with the egg at conception.

How can I maximise my chances of getting pregnant?

Looking at your lifestyle and taking steps to improve it before you start trying to conceive can help to prepare your body for the demands of pregnancy and pave the way for the conception of a healthy baby.

- Eat a varied healthy diet. A nutritious diet can ensure that all your body's cells are healthy and ready to conceive.
- Maintain a healthy weight. In women weight can influence hormone levels and affect fertility. Being overweight (which may be linked to polycystic ovary syndrome) has also been linked to an increased risk of diabetes and heart disease. Having too little body fat eg due to excessive dieting or exercise, can also disturb the normal fertility cycle.
- Take regular exercise. Benefits include improving the strength and capacity of your heart and lungs (essential for the demands of carrying a baby), improving mood and helping you relax.
- Get a sexual health check. Infections of the reproductive tract, such as chlamydia and gonorrhoea, can affect fertility (see p.46). It is worth you and your partner visiting a local genito-urinary clinic to be checked for any 'silent' sexually transmitted infections so they can be treated before you start to try to conceive.
- Moderate your alcohol intake (see below).
- Avoid recreational drugs. It's wise to steer clear of recreational drugs if you are trying to conceive. Cannabis can interfere with ovulation and can also lower the sperm count. When used during pregnancy, it can lead to premature birth. Ecstasy can activate latent infections or problems in the female reproductive tract and cocaine crosses the placenta.

Could the timing of sex increase my likelihood of conception?

Your best chance of conceiving lies in having sex at the time your cervical mucus is most receptive to sperm – that is, one or two days before ovulation. Timing sex to coincide precisely with ovulation is not usually that effective and can put a terrible strain on your relationship. Instead, having sex regularly – say every two to four days – can substantially increase your chances of conceiving, given that it is only possible to conceive on three or four days each month. Research shows that couples having sex three times a month take an average of 15 months to conceive, compared to couples who have sex more than 15 times a month who take just three and a half.

Will abstaining from sex make conception more likely?
Once produced, sperm's quality and motility deteriorate so abstinence could actually decrease your likelihood of conception.

Could stress stop me from conceiving?
Most fertility experts insist that stress does not cause infertility. However, there is no doubt that hormones are sensitive to the effects of anxiety. In fact, according to the American Society for Reproductive Medicine, some studies suggest that stress can cause fallopian tube spasm in women and decrease sperm production in men. Consider good time-management and other stress-reduction techniques such as exercise, relaxation, yoga and meditation.

Could giving up alcohol increase my chance of conceiving?
The full effects of alcohol on human conception are still undecided. In other animals it is known to reduce levels of sex hormones, inhibit ovulation and interfere with the transport of sperm. Heavy drinking can affect fertility in both women and men. Effects include:
- higher rates of menstrual problems including lack of periods (amenorrhoea), painful periods (dysmenorrhoea) and irregular periods
- a higher incidence of miscarriage, premature and stillbirth and a risk of fetal abnormalities if excessive alcohol is consumed during pregnancy
- a reduction in the ability to manufacture sperm and possible interference with normal structure and movement by inhibiting the metabolism of vitamin A, which is vital for healthy sperm.

What is less certain is what effect, if any, a moderate alcohol intake may have. One Danish research study carried out in 1998 found that even drinking five or fewer drinks a week could affect a woman's chances of conception. However, more recent research has failed to confirm this finding. If you are having problems conceiving, you may wish to have a look at your alcohol consumption and consider cutting down or giving up to see whether it makes a difference.

Recommended limits

Men	3–4 units per day (21–28 units per week).
Women	2–3 units per day (14–21 units per week).
1 unit is	half a pint of beer (normal strength)
	1 small glass of wine (100ml)
	1 measure of spirits (25ml)
	1 measure of sherry (50ml)

Binge drinking heavily one or two days a week is also harmful, even if you remain within your weekly recommended limit. The following levels of drinking are likely to cause harmful effects upon your overall health:

	Men	Women
Moderate Risk	28–49 units/week	21–34 units/week
High Risk	50 or more units/week	35 or more units/week

What about smoking?

There are very good reasons for both you and your partner to quit if you smoke and are trying for a baby. Chemicals in cigarette smoke are poisonous to both eggs and sperm and smoking can affect fertility in both men and women. Smokers take an average of 30 per cent longer to become pregnant than non-smokers and smoking can also reduce the likelihood of conceiving using assisted conception such as in vitro fertilisation (IVF). In fact, it has been found that smoking can reduce your chance of conceiving by 50–70 per cent per cycle. In women undergoing IVF, the proportion of eggs fertilised is some 20 to 30 per cent lower in smokers than in non-smokers. Smoking can also affect sperm production, which may not matter too much in a man with a normal sperm count but in one whose sperm count is lowered may make the difference between conceiving and not conceiving. Smoking is also linked to a higher incidence of miscarriage, stillbirth and low birth weight.

Are there any foods I should include or exclude from my diet?

In order to follow a nutritious, healthy diet, you should make sure you get the following daily: five or more servings of fruit and vegetables, four or five servings of starchy carbohydrates like bread, potatoes and pasta, three servings of milk and dairy products and two servings of meat, fish, pulses or other vegetable proteins. Some preconception advisers recommend taking a vitamin and mineral supplement tailored for pregnant women. However, most orthodox doctors consider this unnecessary unless there is reason to suspect you may have nutritional deficiencies as a result of illness or excessive dieting.

One vitamin that is known to be essential is folic acid – a B vitamin found in green leafy vegetables, oranges, potatoes and fortified foods such as cereals. A shortage of folic acid is linked to a higher incidence of spina bifida and other defects affecting the fetus's developing nervous system. Government guidelines suggest that all women who may get pregnant should consume 0.4 mg a day before conception and for the first 12 weeks of pregnancy.

Can we still drink tea and coffee?

A moderate intake of tea and coffee should do you no harm. However, too much caffeine (found in coffee, tea, cola-type drinks, other soft drinks and 'alcopops') may affect sperm motility (movement) and in women may lower levels of the hormone prolactin, produced by the pituitary to stimulate milk production after birth. High prolactin levels (hyperprolactinaemia) can inhibit ovulation. If you consume more than six cups of caffeinated drinks a day, it may be worth trying to cut down or switching to decaffeinated alternatives.

Can too much soya prevent conception?

Soya (milk, tofu and other products) is a source of phytoestrogens, weak oestrogenic compounds found in plant-based foods. Other sources include linseeds and pulses such as chickpeas. There is evidence that phytoestrogens lengthen the first phase of the menstrual cycle, leading to fewer cycles, and may also affect sperm production. However, some nutritional practitioners argue that phytoestrogen-rich foods can help to make the menstrual cycle more regular and increase the chances of conception. It is worth discussing the issue with your doctor to find out what the latest thinking is.

Understanding fertility problems

Medically, infertility is defined as an inability to conceive within one year of having regular sex without using contraception. To produce a baby, a healthy sperm must meet and fuse with a healthy egg at a favourable time for conception to occur and the egg must then successfully implant in the uterus. If anything consistently goes wrong at any point in this process, infertility can be the result.

What causes infertility?

In women the most common causes include:

- anovulation caused by medical conditions such as polycystic ovary syndrome (PCOS) or premature menopause
- blocked fallopian tubes caused by pelvic inflammatory disease or scarring from endometriosis
- cervical mucus problems preventing sperm from swimming into the uterus

In men common causes include:

- poor-quality sperm due to ageing or reduction of testosterone
- insufficient quantity of sperm (poor sperm count)
- problems with sustaining an erection and with ejaculation, possibly caused by illness or certain medications
- damage or blockage of the epididymis due to infection or scarring

The combined effect of your and your partner's fertility may also present a problem, eg if your partner's sperm count is low this may not matter all that much if you are ovulating regularly. However, if your partner's sperm count is low and you are also not ovulating regularly, you may have difficulty conceiving.

Is infertility the same as subfertility?

Strictly speaking, infertility is a complete inability to conceive. In fact, very few couples are truly infertile. Most who seek help are actually subfertile – that is, they have problems that make conception unlikely without medical help. The term also includes women who conceive but have trouble carrying a baby to term because of recurrent miscarriage.

What are primary and secondary infertility?

Primary infertility is the inability to conceive at all. Secondary infertility is the inability to conceive or maintain a pregnancy after previously having had one or more children. The term is also applied to women who have had one or more miscarriages or stillbirths. Secondary infertility is even more common than primary infertility. It is estimated that between 2 and 10 per cent of all couples have primary infertility, while another 10 to 25 per cent have secondary infertility.

Are the causes of primary and secondary infertility the same?

Many of the causes are the same. However, there may also be factors to do with a previous pregnancy or delivery or things that have happened since then. These include:

- infection or damage while giving birth, or while undergoing miscarriage or termination of pregnancy
- complications caused by pelvic surgery
- the development of certain acute or chronic illnesses eg thyroid problems
- certain undiagnosed medical conditions
- a change of partner
- a less active sex life since the time when you conceived previously
- increased age, especially if there has been a big gap between having your previous child and trying to conceive again

How common is infertility?

Infertility is surprisingly common. According to the World Health Organisation, between 60 and 80 million couples are infertile worldwide. In the UK, one in six couples is affected. In fact, apart from pregnancy, difficulty conceiving is possibly the most common reason for people between 20 and 45 to seek medical advice. Although in the past infertility used to be thought of as the woman's problem, it is now recognised that fertility problems affect men and women equally.

Is the number of people who are infertile on the increase?

The number of couples seeking help from fertility specialists has increased over the past 15 years. However, experts don't believe this is due to any major change in prevalence but to a number of other factors.

- Infertility has a higher profile than it had in the past and couples are more willing to seek help and talk about their problems.
- Fewer babies are available for adoption and so couples are more likely to seek medical assistance rather than choosing to adopt.
- A woman aged between 35 and 44 is twice as likely to have fertility problems as a woman aged 30 to 34 and the current trend is for couples to delay having children until their 30s or even 40s.
- Some research suggests that sperm counts have dropped in the last 50 years, although others have not confirmed this. It is possible that they have not actually fallen but that investigative procedures have become more rigorous and accurate.

How long should it take to conceive?

For a healthy, fertile couple, the chance of conception in any one month is only around 20 per cent – incidentally around the same as for IVF. Given Nature's relative inefficiency, it is not at all unusual to have unprotected sex for several months before becoming pregnant. Approximately 70 per cent of couples do succeed in conceiving within six months of stopping contraception; 85 per cent conceive within a year and 95 per cent within two years. Because of this, most doctors will not investigate infertility unless a couple has been trying for at least a year, unless there are specific reasons for suspecting a problem.

How does my age affect my chances of conception?

In women, natural fertility gradually declines from the mid-20s onwards. This means that your chances of becoming pregnant decrease with every year that passes, while your risk of miscarrying if you do conceive also increases. As a rule, a woman of 35 is half as fertile as one of 25 and a woman of 40 half as fertile as one of 35.

Why does female fertility decline so fast?

At birth all your eggs are already present in your ovaries. As you grow older, and particularly as menopause approaches, the number of follicles (fluid-filled sacs in which the eggs develop) and eggs in the ovaries diminish,as does their quality. This may be because of accumulated damage, environmental assaults or because the female body has a 'sorting' mechanism that ensures that the best quality eggs are released earlier in life.

At menopause, the ovaries stop producing eggs, menstrual activity decreases and eventually ceases, and the body decreases the production of the female hormones, estrogen and progesterone. After this transitional period, the supply of eggs runs out altogether, although the uterus is still capable of accommodating a fetus – which is why some women who have gone through the menopause are still able to bear a child using a donor egg. Although the menopause is the time at which you stop having periods, it is preceded by the perimenopause (the two- to 15-year span before menopause, during which time a woman experiences changes due to declining levels of estrogen and progesterone). During this time, you may still be menstruating but no longer ovulating. The precise time at which your eggs run out is genetically programmed, so if your mother had an early menopause you are also likely to do so.

What about my partner's age?

As the many famous examples of older fathers from Picasso to Michael Douglas show, men retain their potential fertility for longer than women. Recent research suggests that men's fertility also takes a downward turn with age, showing that in men over 25, the likelihood of their partner conceiving within six or 12 months was lower than for men under 25. This then declined progressively with age. Reasons may include lower levels of sexual activity or problems maintaining an erection (perhaps as a result of heart disease or medications used to treat other health problems). By the age of 55 there is a higher risk of passing on a chromosomal abnormality such as Down's syndrome. For these reasons, the HFEA recommends that sperm donors must be under 45 unless the sperm is for their own partner or in exceptional circumstances.

Are there any medical problems associated with infertility?

The following current or previous medical problems can affect fertility.

In women:

- **Previous pelvic or abdominal surgery** eg for cancer, appendicitis or removal of an ovarian cyst. This may have caused scar tissue to form and block the fallopian tubes.
- **Previous pelvic infections** can also cause scarring of the ovaries so that follicles are unable to develop properly.

- **Polycystic ovary syndrome (PCOS)** Between 5 and 10 per cent of women between late adolescence and the menopause have polycystic ovary syndrome, which is one of the major causes of infertility. PCOS is characterised by excessive levels of testosterone and abnormal levels of LH. The ovaries contain many small follicles which have stopped growing. Symptoms include acne, increased body hair (or hair thinning), being overweight, heavy or absent periods and failure to ovulate (anovulation).
- **Thyroid problems** An underactive thyroid (hypothyroidism) can affect the quality of eggs released and also increase the risk of miscarriage. If you go for fertility treatment, your thyroid hormone levels will be routinely checked.
- **Diabetes** Although diabetes is not directly linked to infertility, autoimmune diseases – of which type 1 diabetes (childhood onset) is one – can increase the risk of early menopause (premature ovarian failure). This, in turn, can cause fertility problems.
- **Inflammatory bowel diseases,** such as Crohn's disease or surgery for ulcerative colitis, may affect fertility.
- **Epilepsy** In one study, fertility rates were 33 per cent lower among women with epilepsy than among those without. This may be due to some anti-epilepsy drugs.
- **Treatment for cancer** Both chemotherapy and radiation therapy often cause irreversible sterility. While an FSH level after therapy can often indicate whether fertility may be possible, a discussion about fertility potential should have preceded any treatment.

In men:
- **Orchitis (inflammation of the testes)** This can be a complication of a virus such as mumps, which can affect sperm production. When caused by a previous bacterial infection, it can result in scarring and blockage of the vas deferens and epididymis.
- **Previous surgery** Surgery to correct a hernia, undescended testicles or testicular torsion may have damaged the tubes of the reproductive system or restricted blood flow to the testes.
- **Treatment for cancer** Both chemotherapy and radiation therapy often cause irreversible sterility. If infertility is expected after a particular regimen of therapy, the patient often has the option to provide semen specimens that can be frozen for later use.

What about any medication I'm taking?

It is best to avoid all but essential medication if you are trying to get pregnant. If you have a chronic condition (such as diabetes, epilepsy or rheumatoid arthritis) for which you must take regular medication, you should consult your doctor before you try to conceive, as your medication may need to be changed. If you are taking any other medications regularly – whether prescribed, over-the-counter or herbal remedies – you should check with your GP, pharmacist or local fertility clinic. The following drugs can decrease fertility, although fertility should return to normal when the medication is stopped.

In women

- Psychiatric medications, such as some tranquillisers and sedatives, can cause excessive production by the pituitary of the milk-producing hormone prolactin, which blocks ovulation.
- Anti-nausea drugs such as metoclopramide can also raise prolactin levels.
- Anti-inflammatory drugs and drugs used to treat arthritis, such as indomethacin, naproxen and diclofenac can block ovulation.
- Painkillers, such as aspirin and paracetamol, may cause problems if taken in high doses, particularly if taken mid-cycle.
- Acetaminophen may reduce oestrogen and LH levels.
- Sodium valproate – PCOS may be more common in women with epilepsy and some evidence suggests that this common anti-seizure drug may also induce the syndrome.

In men

- Sulphasalazine, used to treat inflammatory bowel diseases such as Crohn's disease. Men taking this drug can develop a reduced sperm count and so become infertile, although this effect ceases when the drug is stopped.
- Anti-hypertensive drugs to treat high blood pressure, eg beta-blockers and captopril, can cause erectile problems in some men.
- Anti-malarial drugs can reduce sperm counts.
- Pain killers, eg aspirin (if over-used), can also lower sperm counts.
- Chemotherapy is likely to damage sperm production and you should talk to your consultant about sperm banking before treatment begins.
- Anabolic steroids used by some body-builders are associated with male infertility.

How can I tell if I'm ovulating?

The first thing you need to understand is how hormones rise and fall at different times of the fertility cycle. The second is to learn how to apply this understanding to your own body. Doing so will not only increase your chances of conceiving, but will also help you to feel more in control of your body when you are trying to conceive.

Generally, if you are having regular periods you are almost certainly ovulating. As a result of changes in the reproductive organs and the rest of your body caused by fluctuating hormones, you can learn to recognise clues as to when ovulation is happening.

- **Testing basal body temperature (BBT)** Body temperature in a healthy young person generally falls within 97.5°F (36.4°C) to 98.9°F (37.2°C). About 24 hours before ovulation, body temperature falls under the influence of LH. After ovulation, body temperature rises slightly (by about 0.2 degrees) under the influence of progesterone. Testing BBT is one of the mainstays of 'natural family planning' and temperature charts are available from GPs, family planning advisers and in many books on natural family planning and infertility. Because ovulation can only be detected in retrospect and temperature can also be affected by other factors such as drinking or infection, temperature charting is a fairly hit and miss method of determining ovulation. With more sophisticated methods available eg ovulation predictor kits (see p.25), BBT testing has become less popular. What it can do, however, is help you understand your own fertility cycle.

- **Detecting changes in cervical mucus** Mucus produced by the cells of the cervix changes in texture and consistency throughout the menstrual cycle under the influence of hormones. You may be aware of this as variations in normal 'vaginal discharge' throughout your cycle. Immediately following menstruation, the mucus is scanty, thick and 'pasty' in consistency making it hard for sperm to swim in it. A couple of days before ovulation the mucus becomes more copious, clear and stretchy in consistency rather like raw egg white, enabling sperm to swim through the opening of the cervix and into the uterus. Once ovulation has taken place, the mucus becomes unreceptive to sperm. Becoming aware of these changes can help you to work out the most favourable time to conceive.

- **Detecting changes in the position and consistency of the cervix**
  The cervix is the gateway to the uterus. You can feel it as a firmish 'knuckle' at the end of your vagina if you insert your forefinger and middle finger. During the menstrual cycle it changes in position and consistency under the influence of hormones. Just after a menstrual period it is firm and high in the vagina. Towards ovulation it softens slightly, drops down lower in the vagina and its opening (the os) becomes slightly wider to allow sperm to swim up into the uterus.
- **Other signs of ovulation** Once you become attuned to your own fertility cycle you may become aware of other, sometimes quite subtle, signs of ovulation such as changes in appetite, skin and hair and desire for sex. Some women experience a sharp pain called Mittelschmerz mid-cycle around the time of ovulation, while others experience more vague abdominal pain.

What is the Persona system and can it help me to conceive?

Persona was designed as a form of contraception. It measures FSH and LH levels in order to predict when ovulation is likely. It consists of a small plastic box and urine dipsticks (like those in pregnancy testing kits) that you use to check the first urine of the morning for hormone levels. The stick is inserted into the Persona which 'reads' the hormone levels and indicates if unprotected sex is safe. Details of your menstrual cycle are programmed into the device's memory, allowing it to predict 'safe' days, taking around three months to recognise your personal cycle. You could also use Persona in reverse to aid conception but it is expensive to buy (£64.99 plus £9.95 a month for the sticks).

Are there any fertility kits that my partner and I can use?

At the time of writing, a 'his and hers' fertility test kit 'Fertell' is about to be launched in the UK. It measures FSH levels, showing how well your ovaries are working, and includes a test designed to measure the amount of sperm your partner is producing and its activity. The kit contains a tube of synthetic mucus up which sperm should swim. After a short period it will indicate whether sufficient numbers of sperm have swum through. It is designed to give an early indication of any potential problems with the male partner. Whilst it can't diagnose all causes of male fertility, it will identify many.

Getting help

If you have been trying for a baby unsuccessfully for some time, you may begin to suspect that you and your partner may have fertility problems. As we have already seen, there are some measures you can take to check if you are ovulating. However, the only way to be certain is to have investigations to assess your fertility.

How long should I try to conceive before I think there might be a problem?

There's no simple answer to this. Generally, you should seek medical help if you have been trying to conceive unsuccessfully for at least a year. However, because of the steep natural decline in fertility after the age of 40, the time it may take to investigate infertility problems, long waiting times for treatment and the age ceiling often applied to NHS funding, many fertility experts recommend seeking help after six months if you are over 35.

When to seek help

You are a woman and you

- are aged 35 and have not conceived within six months
- suffer from pelvic inflammatory disease (PID)
- have infrequent or absent periods or have been diagnosed with polycystic ovary syndrome (PCOS)
- have had one or more previous miscarriages or ectopic pregnancy
- have had severe appendicitis or abdominal surgery
- have had a positive test for a sexually transmitted infection eg chlamydia or gonorrhoea, both of which can cause PID
- find sex painful – this may be a sign of endometriosis

You are a man and you

- have had an infection of the testes (orchitis) eg caused by mumps
- have had surgery for undescended testicles
- have been treated for sexually transmitted diseases eg gonorrhoea
- have sexual problems such as premature ejaculation or difficulty achieving or sustaining an erection
- have a job that exposes you to radiation or industrial chemicals

You and your partner
- are under 30 but have not used contraception for 18 months.

Are there any tests I can perform on myself before I consider going to see the doctor?

It is advisable to seek the help of your GP, have proper medical investigations and get into the system as quickly as possible. You may still want to check for yourself if you are ovulating by observing signs or buying a predictor kit and using it for a couple of months.

Will it matter if we don't seek help straightaway?

Undergoing tests and investigations for infertility can be time-consuming so it's important to seek medical advice as soon as you suspect there may be a problem. Delay in seeking help may affect your treatment options and/or hinder the chance of them being effective. Many couples find it hard to accept that they may have a fertility problem and carry on trying month after month without seeking medical help. Others delay seeking help because they fear being asked intimate questions about their sex lives or because they are worried about the investigations and treatments that they may have to undergo. These feelings are extremely normal. Your GP and the staff at the fertility clinic are used to dealing with people who have these worries and should give you all the advice and information you need to decide whether to go ahead with treatment.

Where should we seek help in the first instance?

Initially you should make an appointment to see your GP. They can perform some simple tests and refer you to your local hospital or a specialist fertility clinic for further investigations if necessary.

If we decide to use a private fertility clinic will a referral from the GP be necessary?

You can self-refer yourself to a private doctor without having a letter from your GP. Simply phone the clinic or the specialist's consulting rooms and ask to make an appointment. However, even if you intend to take the private route, it's probably a good idea to get at least some initial tests carried out by your GP in case you have a straightforward problem that can easily be solved.

My partner is reluctant to come with me. Does it matter?

Traditionally infertility was viewed as a woman's problem and it was the woman who sought help. However, fertility problems affect men and women equally, so both of you will need to be investigated. The Royal College of Obstetricians and Gynaecologists recommends that people in a relationship should be seen as a couple. If your partner is reluctant to come with you, it may help to go for a preliminary consultation alone and then attend a subsequent appointment together, or your partner may feel more comfortable making a separate appointment to see the GP.

There are things in my past I don't want my partner to know about. Should I make a separate appointment?

You or your partner may have things in your past – a sexually transmitted diseases or a previous termination – that you haven't discussed with each other and wish to keep private. You should be able to be examined separately and talk confidentially to your doctor.

What is the GP likely to do?

The GP should give you some advice on how to maximise your chances of conception. They should also carry out an initial assessment of your fertility and do some preliminary basic tests. They may then either suggest that you keep trying for a few more months, or refer you to a specialist clinic.

What questions will the GP ask us?

The GP should take full medical histories from both you and your partner to see if they provide any clues to your problems. It is important to be honest so that the doctor can get as full a picture as possible of your fertility and any factors that may be affecting it.

You will both be asked to provide details about your lifestyle, overall health, any previous or current medical problems, any regular medication and your menstrual cycle, and you will need to give details of any previous pregnancies and existing children. Also, you need to tell the GP about your sex life and any difficulties there. Your partner will be specifically asked about any problems affecting his genito-urinary system (eg undescended testes), whether or not he has had mumps, and whether he has problems having an erection.

Will the doctor examine me?

This will depend on the GP. At the very least they will look for signs (such as excess hair or acne) which can indicate PCOS. They may perform a vaginal examination and palpate your abdomen to check for fibroids, ovarian cysts or tenderness (which can be a sign of endometriosis) and check for evidence of any vaginal infection that needs to be treated. However, not all GPs will do this.

Will the doctor examine my partner?

Again this will depend on the GP. A physical examination will include checking your partner's penis for any abnormalities or inflammation, and the size and consistency of his testicles. Small, soft testicles can be a sign that sperm formation is damaged. They will check for varicocele (varicose veins around the testicle, see p.64), found in a quarter of men being assessed for infertility. They will also feel for any potentially cancerous lumps (although testicular cancer is rare, it is the most common form of cancer in men aged 15 to 45).

Will the GP perform any initial investigations?

The GP will usually perform a few simple tests, likely to include:

Blood tests

- **Ovulation check test** Irregular ovulation is the most common problem affecting fertility. A blood sample is taken to check the level of progesterone which rises following ovulation (see p.11). The sample needs to be taken seven days before your next expected period – if taken too early or late, progesterone levels will be too low to be meaningful. If the result suggests you are not ovulating, the test should be repeated. Ovulation is commonly irregular in the first few months after coming off the contraceptive pill, but usually rights itself without any treatment.

- **Rubella (German measles)** All women planning a pregnancy should be screened for rubella. Although a fairly mild illness, rubella can damage the unborn baby if contracted before the twelfth week of pregnancy. The GP should check to see whether you have rubella antibodies (showing you have had rubella or been injected against it) by taking a blood sample, and if not, you will be offered immunisation. You should not try to get pregnant for a month afterwards.

- **Other conditions** If your menstrual cycle is less than 21 days or more than 35, the doctor may test your blood to check for hormonal conditions such as polycystic ovary syndrome or premature menopause. Blood tests may also be taken to establish your FSH levels – FSH levels of 10 or more may suggest premature menopause.

Semen analysis (sperm count)

The doctor will normally ask your partner to supply at least one sample of semen which will be sent for laboratory analysis to check for the number of sperm, their motility and volume. If the sample shows few or no sperm, the test will be repeated – usually some three or four weeks later – and if the result is still the same, the GP should refer you for specialist investigation (see p.52).

It is a good idea to ask your GP if the laboratory the semen sample is sent to would be the same one you would be referred to if further investigation is recommended. If not, you will have to repeat the test. You might also want to check if the laboratory takes part in the UK National External Quality Assessment Scheme (UK NEQAS). This scheme gives objective information and advice to clinical laboratories on the quality of their analytical and interpretative performance.

Do's and don'ts of providing a sperm sample

Do

- abstain from sex for two to three days before providing the sample
- produce the sample by masturbation
- collect the sample in a wide-mouthed sterile plastic specimen pot (the GP should provide one)
- deliver the sample to the lab as quickly as possible (within an hour). There may be facilities on site for collecting a sample
- make sure the sample is kept at between 15°C and 38°C during transportation

Don't

- use coitus interruptus (withdrawal before ejaculation) to produce the sample – it's not usually possible to withdraw quickly enough to ensure all sperm are caught and female secretions can interfere with results
- use condoms or lubricant gels as these may interfere with the quality of the sperm.

Urine tests

The GP may ask you and your partner to supply a urine sample to check for chlamydia, a major cause of blocked fallopian tubes (see p.46). If the GP doesn't do this test, it should be done at a genito-urinary clinic or the specialist fertility clinic.

Will the GP suggest doing anything before referring us to a specialist?

If your GP cannot find a specific problem, they may suggest you try to conceive for a few more months before they refer you. They may also give you advice on how to maximise your chances of conception, such as stopping smoking, cutting down on alcohol, eating a healthy diet and exercising. If your partner's sperm count is poor, the GP will advise him to wear loose-fitting underwear and trousers. Also, if he works in a job that exposes him to conditions that may cause the testes to overheat (long-distance lorry driving, for example), he may be advised to visit an occupational health specialist, who will advise him on what aspects of his work may be contributing to any potential fertility problems. He will also be told to avoid other activities that may raise the heat of his testes, for example saunas. Research suggests that exposure to hazardous chemicals and solvents lowers sperm count.

I don't want to 'go away and keep trying' – what can I do?

Many women who have had fertility treatment advise that it is best to get help as soon as possible rather than wait. However, if your GP has advised you to come back again in a few months' time, and you are unhappy with this recommendation, you can change your GP (see below) or refer yourself directly to a fertility clinic privately.

My GP doesn't seem very interested. Is there anything I can do?

Most GPs have a heavy work-load and don't have much time to spend with each patient. Some GPs have a strong interest in infertility while others may be inexperienced or downright unsympathetic. However, your GP can be an invaluable source of support and information in your journey through the infertility maze and, if you are undergoing fertility treatment, may be able to write you an NHS prescription for some of your drugs. If your GP seems uninterested, it is worth looking around to find one who is more sympathetic. CHILD or ISSUE may have a local group in your area who can advise you on local GPs with an interest in infertility. To change your GP all you need to do is to take your medical card to the new surgery, although there may be waiting lists for popular surgeries, so it is a good idea to get hold of the practice leaflet and check beforehand.

My GP has suggested I keep a temperature chart. Is this useful ?
Some GPs suggest keeping a temperature chart so you can time sex to coincide with ovulation (see p.24). Provided you are having regular sex two to three times a week, there should be no need to keep a temperature chart or to use an ovulation prediction kit.

What will happen when I've seen my GP?
Once your GP has the results of the various tests they should be able to give you a preliminary assessment of the nature of your problem. What happens next will depend on the following:
• If your medical history, examination and test results were normal and you have been trying for less than 18 months, the GP may suggest trying longer before referring you to a specialist.
• Your doctor may refer you to a gynaecologist at your local hospital for further investigations and possibly treatment (see below). This will usually be funded by the NHS.
• If your GP thinks that you need IVF or ICSI, they may refer you to a local NHS unit that provides these treatments or, if you want private treatment, they will refer you to a private clinic.

Will fertility treatment always be necessary?
Sometimes subfertility can be solved by making a few simple lifestyle changes and making sure you have sex regularly and often. This can lead to conception without the need for any further treatment.

I've heard that GPs can prescribe fertility drugs but my GP has not offered this. Why not?
Until fairly recently, if the semen analysis was normal and ovulation failure appeared to be the main problem, GPs used to be able to prescribe drugs that would induce ovulation. Recently, however, concerns have been raised about the long-term effects of these drugs

(see p.69). Therefore, if you appear to have an ovulatory problem, the doctor will refer you to a specialist for further investigation and treatment. However, if you have been prescribed drugs to induce ovulation by a fertility specialist, it is worth contacting your GP, who may be able to write you an NHS prescription for them.

When should the GP refer us to a specialist?

The doctor should refer you without delay if:

- you are 35 or older.
- your menstrual cycle is less than 21 days or longer than 35 days.
- the level of progesterone in your ovulation test is less than 20 nmol/l, which may mean that you are not ovulating.
- you have previously had an ectopic pregnancy, pelvic infection, endometriosis or any abnormalities in the anatomy or structure of your reproductive organs.
- you and your partner have not conceived within three years of stopping using contraception. In this case, your likelihood of conceiving without medical help falls to 5 per cent.

What questions should I ask my GP about referral to a fertility specialist?

Your GP will probably have no more than six minutes to answer your questions, so it is worth thinking about what information would be most useful to you:

- What clinics and treatments are available in this area? See the back of this guide for details on costs and how to choose a clinic.
- Is there a particular clinic you refer patients to and if so why?
- How long will we have to wait to be referred to a specialist centre?
- Is there anything we can do to avoid unnecessary delay?
- Are the tests and treatments needed available on the NHS?
- If not, what are the costs associated with tests or treatments?
- Will you support us by prescribing any drugs needed or covering the cost of tests?
- Do you have written or other information on the tests and procedures I and my partner will have?
- Is there anyone I can talk to about tests and treatment?
- Can you refer me to a counsellor with whom I can discuss my feelings?

How can we avoid delays and ensure a prompt diagnosis?

One of the most frustrating things for couples treated for infertility is the delay in diagnosis and referral. This is very common if you are using the NHS. If you feel you are having to wait too long, there are several approaches you can try:

- Call the appointments department of the clinic to which you have been referred to see if there have been any cancellations and ask whether it may be possible to schedule an earlier appointment.
- If there are particularly pressing reasons for you to be seen quickly (eg your age, or a known medical condition that is likely to make it hard to conceive), your GP may be able to help by sending a letter emphasising the need for an early consultation.
- If you have the funds, you may be able to make a private appointment for an initial consultation, even if you want to have some of your subsequent treatment on the NHS.
- If you've been referred to a general hospital rather than a specialist unit on the NHS, you can see if other hospitals in your area have a shorter waiting list for appointments (but only if treatment via your health authority or PCT is available at these other hospitals).
- Keeping accurate details of your own medical history that you can show to the doctor may speed up diagnosis and treatment. Include details of your menstrual cycle, together with names of all doctors you have seen or been referred to, and the dates of appointments, tests and their results. Also note medications prescribed, their dosage and how long you took them for.

Am I too old for fertility treatment?

Both the number and quality of eggs deteriorates as women approach the menopause and, although this decline is gradual at first, it accelerates after the age of 35. The doctor should do FSH blood tests (see p.48) to check your 'ovarian reserve'. These are designed to measure hormones indicating ovarian function – that is your ability to produce the hormones needed to conceive and fertilise eggs. If you are found to have little ovarian reserve, you may want to think about egg donation (see p.123).

Can I be refused treatment on the grounds of my age?

Most consultants do have age criteria as to whom they will treat. Between the ages of 35 and 40 you still have a high chance of success using assisted conception. After 40, fertility begins to decline rapidly and your chances of conceiving will be severely limited unless you choose to use donor eggs or more complicated forms of treatment.

The age after which fertility specialists may not offer treatment varies tremendously. If a consultant at one clinic won't treat you, you may find one somewhere else who will. Some will not take women over 35; others draw the line at 40 or 45. You are extremely unlikely to find a consultant to treat you after you have passed the age of 50, as your chances of success are minimal and the risk of complications is greatly increased. However, it is very important that you feel you can trust your consultant to advise you responsibly, rather than spending thousands of pounds on treatments that have little or no chance of success.

Are there any ways I can judge what my chances of success are likely to be?

Your chances of conception are greater if:

- you have recently conceived and/or given birth.
- there is a treatable reason for your problem, such as tubal blockage. In this case, poor egg quality is less likely to be the main reason for your failure to conceive.
- you have not experienced premenopausal symptoms, such as changes in the length of your menstrual cycle and/or the pattern of your periods, vaginal dryness, hot flushes.
- tests for ovarian reserve are normal.

Your chances of conception are less if:

- you have been trying to conceive without success for over three years.
- you have unexplained infertility.
- your ovarian reserve suggests you are approaching the menopause.
- your menstrual cycle has changed in the past few years. For example, your cycles have become shorter or more irregular.

Choosing a clinic

If you are being treated on the NHS, the clinic you go to will be determined by which hospitals provide services to your PCT (with whom they will have a contract). Lack of funding and long waiting lists mean that many couples have little choice but to fund their own treatment. However, this does at least mean that you can choose which clinic you go to, and it really is worth shopping around. At the back of this guide, we tell you what services are provided by nearly every NHS and private clinic licensed to carry out fertility treatment in the UK. In addition, there are several sources that can help you find and access treatment. CHILD and ISSUE (see p.265 and p.266) both have information on clinics and what you should look for when choosing one. ISSUE's quarterly newsletter contains accounts by people undergoing fertility treatments of their experiences at various clinics, or consult HFEA's free booklet, *The Patient's Guide to DI and IVF Clinics*.

How can we decide between NHS and private treatment?
Your options will depend partly on what funding is available in your area, your age, circumstances and the amount of money you have available. Most NHS clinics offer a full range of basic tests and also provide some treatments eg ovulation induction (see p.68) and tubal surgery (see p.59). However, there may be limits on whether you are eligible for assisted conception. At present, some 80 per cent of assisted conception treatments (such as IVF or ICSI) occur in private clinics. Even clinics that officially offer free NHS assisted conception may charge you if you don't fall within their eligibility criteria.

Can we switch between the NHS and private treatment?
Because the NHS funds some kinds of treatment and not others, it is quite usual for couples to have some of their treatment on the NHS (for example, fertility drug treatment) and then move on to private treatment (for example, IVF). You can choose to leave the NHS and be treated privately at any time.

How much does private treatment cost?

Prices can vary enormously, sometimes by several thousand pounds. Working out the exact costs can be difficult because some clinics offer package deals that include consultation and some tests, while others list the price for each treatment separately. Typically, it costs around £2000 upwards for one cycle of straightforward IVF. If you have had your investigations carried out under the NHS, you won't necessarily have to budget for these, but you will have to budget for costs that may not be included in the package price, such as drugs, or additional procedures that may be required such as assisted hatching (see p.98), plus the cost of freezing and storing embryos and sperm. At the back of this guide, we tell you what each clinic charges for one cycle of IVF and one of IUI, and what is included in these costs. It is also a good idea to request price lists from several different clinics.

Will I get better treatment if I go privately?

Most consultants working in private clinics also work within the NHS so you won't necessarily get better treatment. What you will almost certainly get is faster treatment. This may be a significant consideration if you are over 35 and certainly if you are nearing 40. The environment in which you are seen and treated is also likely to be more comfortable in a private clinic than in most NHS units.

What should I look for when choosing a private clinic?

At the back of this guide, we tell you what to look out for when choosing a clinic and what each clinic provides in terms of treatments and services. It is also a good idea to get the brochures of several clinics for comparison. Some clinics are well established with a good reputation and a great deal of expertise, others will be newer and relatively untested. The reputation of a clinic and its director is important – newer clinics are not necessarily inferior – sometimes they will have been founded by consultants who have gained their experience in better known clinics. The location of the clinic and how easy it is to get to is another important factor, as you may have to visit at inconvenient times (such as the middle of the night for an hCG injection – see p.73) for certain tests or procedures. Another key factor is the atmosphere – you will probably have to make a great many visits there over an extended period of time, so it is important that you feel the clinic is comfortable and welcoming, as well as efficient. The clinic should also produce clearly written literature about itself and its treatments. In terms of staffing the clinic should have:

- consultants (specialist doctors), trained in the investigation and treatment of female and male infertility.
- nurses, specially trained in infertility.
- urologists, doctors specialising in the urinary system (as this is closely linked to the reproductive system in men).
- embryologists, specialists in the development of gametes (eggs and sperm) and fertilised eggs.
- counsellors, to offer help and support at every stage of treatment.

The clinic should also have a laboratory with facilities for testing and analysing blood, urine and semen samples. Ideally, consultant anaesthetists should administer any general anaesthetics required.

When we're looking for an assisted conception unit (ACU), should we go for the one with the highest live birth rate?

It seems apparently simple to choose a clinic or ACU with a high live birth rate, just as you might choose a hotel with the highest star rating. After all, what you want is a live baby! But – and it's a big but – the live birth rate in itself isn't as reliable a guide as you might imagine. Birth rates can be affected by:

- patient age – clinics that tend to treat younger women may have a better live birth rate than ones treating older patients, as assisted conception is more likely to be successful in younger women.
- encouraging the use of donated eggs and sperm at an early stage. Using donor eggs (which come from younger women) has a higher success rate even in women over 38.
- the amount of cycles involving patients with a history of unsuccessful treatment or unexplained infertility.

For these reasons, the live birth rate should never be your sole criterion for choosing a clinic. It is far more important to look at its reputation, staff expertise, organisation and how sensitively it meets its patients needs, as well as considering practical aspects eg distance from your home. If you have a particular problem, you may consider looking for a consultant with specialist knowledge in this area. Some clinics publish their pregnancy and birth rates by type of fertility problem, so these are worth looking into.

Questions to ask about success rates

- What are your live birth rates for people with my condition? Ask for birth rates for the latest year and the one before – if the figures are significantly different, ask the clinic to explain why.
- What are your live birth rates for people of my age?
- How many treatment cycles did the clinic carry out last year? This can show how busy it is, which together with staff numbers may help you assess the level of personal care available to you.
- What is the egg fertilisation rate? This may give you an indication of how skilled the unit's embryologist is, especially when performing more specialised techniques such as ICSI.
- How many embryos do you usually replace? (The HFEA stipulates a maximum of two per cycle, three in exceptional cases).
- What is the percentage of positive pregnancy tests and does this include the number of miscarriages?
- What is the success rate for frozen embryos? This is a fairly new technique and not provided by all fertility units.

Should we visit the unit before going ahead?

Most clinics send out written information, or have glossy brochures and sites on the Net. However, there's no real substitute for visiting yourself and getting a feel for the clinic and whether you would feel comfortable there. Many clinics have open days, others will be happy to show you around and arrange for you to meet some of the staff. It's a good idea to go with your partner, a friend or relative so you can compare your impressions. Points to note include:

- General ambience: whether the place is clean and efficient.
- The staff: whether they seem to work well together; if they seem in control or stressed and rushed; whether you feel they would really listen to you and give you the time you need; whether they would be honest in answering your questions even where you might not like the answer, or if there is no definitive answer.
- The tone of the clinic: whether it is formal or informal, will you be encouraged to call staff by their Christian names and how comfortable do you feel with this?
- Convenience: if the clinic is not near your home, where will you stay? Will the clinic be able to accommodate you for appointment times, especially if you live further away?

What questions should I ask when choosing a clinic?

Treatment procedures can vary between different clinics, for example, the frequency of tests and drug regimens. Try to find out the following information before your first appointment:

- What treatments do you offer? How long will I have to wait for treatment? This is especially important if you are older and/or hoping for NHS funding. You don't want to reach the end of the waiting list only to find you are no longer eligible for funding.

- How long has the unit been established? Do the specialists have special expertise or research interests in any particular technique?

- Will I be able to see the same doctor every time? Continuity of care helps you feel that you are more than just a number. If care under one consultant is not available, there may be a named nurse system or care within a small team, eg two doctors and two nurses. If so, ask if it is possible to meet them at the start of treatment.

- Will I be able to see a female consultant if I want to?

- What proportion of the women you treat are over 35/40?

- What is the cancellation rate for treatment cycles? A low rate may indicate that the unit generally treats fairly straightforward cases, which may also be reflected in an apparently high success rate. High cancellation rates may suggest that it takes on more difficult-to-treat cases, or that it takes on too many patients who are unlikely to succeed.

- Are freezing facilities offered for unused embros/eggs?

- What counselling facilities are available? Is there a dedicated counsellor available at all times? Will this person be independent (ie not involved with my medical treatment)? Will I have to pay for this? (See p.150 for more information on counselling.)

- How much do treatments cost? What other costs are likely to be involved?

- Will I have to pay for initial investigations or will you accept results from investigations carried out elsewhere?

- Will I have to buy drugs from the clinic? Cheaper drugs may be available via your GP or from private drug companies (see p.164).

- How will I be expected to pay and does the clinic have any special payment plans to spread the cost of treatment?

Should I consider going abroad for treatment?

A small number of couples with fertility problems do seek treatment abroad – Spain is currently popular – especially for treatments such as egg donation, where donors are more readily available than they are in the UK. This is because foreign donors can be paid for their eggs and sperm (up to $10,000 in the US), whereas in the UK it is illegal to be paid more than £15 plus expenses. There are fewer restrictions on fertility treatment in some foreign countries than there are in the UK, for example, older women can get treated more easily abroad.

You can also get more information about your donor abroad. In the US, the fact that donors are paid gives the recipients the 'right to know' what they are paying for. In the UK, privacy/data protection laws mean that the recipient has no 'right to know' anything other than essential medical data. If you are considering treatment abroad, you will need to take the following factors into account:

Pros

- Investigations, drugs and treatments unavailable or illegal in the UK may be available abroad (for example, gender selection).
- Some fertility doctors in the US and Europe will treat older women, or transfer more embryos than allowed in the UK.
- Egg donors may be more readily available than in the UK as they can receive payment.
- If you choose a donor from abroad, you may be able to have more information about them than is currently available in the UK.
- If you have been refused treatment in the UK because you are single or in a gay relationship, you may be able to get it abroad.

Cons

- Fertility treatment can take a long time and is notoriously stressful. How will you feel in a foreign country using a different language far from the support of your family or friends?
- Treatment abroad, especially in the US, can be extremely expensive. It is a commercial enterprise with no regulation as to how much donors can be paid or how much you can be charged.
- The HFEA keeps a record of all British egg and sperm donors to help track genetic diseases, regulates how procedures are performed and keeps strict controls on when experimental treatments can be offered to the public. None of these protective measures are in place in the US.

- If more than three embryos are transferred, chances of pregnancy may increase as will the likelihood of multiple pregnancy and birth, with all the attendant risks (see p.112).

Will I be able to get fertility treatment if I am single?

Increasingly, single women are turning to fertility clinics for egg or embryo freezing and donor insemination. Enda McVeigh of the Oxford Fertility Clinic says: 'Women are increasingly getting to about 35 and are worried about their fertility. They want help in having a child, because they have not yet found the right partner.'

The HFEA's code of practice stipulates that all patients seeking fertility treatment are to be assessed according to criteria known as 'welfare of the child'. To be given a treatment licence, a clinic has to consider the welfare of any potential child, including 'the need of that child for a father'. Ultimately, this is open to the interpretation of the clinic. If the NHS is funding your treatment, you may come up against 'couples only' criteria. Private clinics have their own policies, and you should not be turned down simply because you are single.

Are lesbian couples eligible for fertility treatment?

Lesbians are very much in the same boat as single women. You should not be turned down simply on the basis of your sexuality. Again, the 'welfare of the child' rule applies – the HFEA stipulates that 'Centres should take note in their procedures of the importance of a stable and supportive environment for any child produced as a result of treatment.' The Pink Parents website (www.pinkparents.org.uk) gives a list of clinics that, in their experience, are lesbian friendly. Some clinics actively state in their portfolio that they treat single women and lesbians, but the only way to be sure is to ring the clinic and ask about their policy.

What if I'm HIV– or Hep C positive?

Chelsea and Westminster Hospital has one of the largest HIV treatment centres in the UK, and offers assisted conception to patients who are HIV positive. For HIV positive men, special sperm washing techniques will be used. For women, close surveillance, antivirus medication during pregnancy, caesarian delivery and bottle feeding will all minimise the risk of virus transmission to your child.

Defining the problem

If you are having your treatment funded by the NHS, your first appointment with the consultant in charge of your care will take place in an NHS fertility clinic. If you have opted for private treatment, the appointment will either be at the specialist's private consulting rooms (in which case the consultant will refer you to the private hospital, or private unit within an NHS hospital with which they have a contract) or at the private fertility clinic you have chosen.

The session will be devoted to establishing the basic facts about your fertility problems, reviewing any investigations and treatment you have had so far and deciding what further tests you will need to have. The consultant may perform a physical examination to check (or double check) for any abnormalities of your reproductive organs, or this may be arranged for a later date. At the end of the session the consultant will outline the recommend tests and should tell you why they will be done and when, and give details of how to book them.

If I use the NHS, will my GP coordinate things or is it up to me?
Your GP should make your initial appointment with the specialist and, ideally, continue to offer support and information once you start fertility treatment. Once in the hospital system, arrangements for appointments will be made directly with you by the clinic, although your GP should be kept informed of your treatment and may play some part, for example in administering drugs.

Can I refer myself directly to a private clinic?
Most clinics prefer a letter of referral from your GP but you can make an appointment directly with a private clinic. They will ask you for your consent to contact your GP, because they are required by the HFEA to ensure that your GP knows no reason why you might not be suitable for any of the treatments offered. If you don't give consent, you may be refused treatment on the basis that the clinic hasn't been able to obtain sufficient relevant information about you to ensure the 'welfare of the child'.

What questions should I ask the consultant?

It's important to make sure that you have as much information as possible about what your treatment will entail and who will be responsible for your care. Ask the consultant:

- What tests will my partner and I be given and why?
- Who will perform these tests and where will they be carried out?
- How long are we likely to have to wait for testing and results?
- Who will give us the results of the tests? Will they be posted to us or will we come in for an appointment?
- Will the results be conclusive and will any need to be repeated?
- Are any further tests likely to be needed? What are these and what will they show?
- Who will oversee my care? Will it be you? If other consultants are involved, can we meet them before treatment starts?
- If I am having assisted conception and need egg collection or embryo transfer, will I see the same consultant every time? Will these procedures be done by a consultant, embryologist or a nurse? (If you haven't seen the facilities at the clinic, you should find out where the embryology lab is in relation to the operating theatre – ideally, they should be as close together as possible. You should also ask to meet the embryologist along with the other members of staff who will be involved with your care.)
- Will I have a dedicated specialist nurse to support me during my treatment? Does the clinic have a support group?
- How might I contact you if I have any queries/problems?

What information should I take with me and what questions will the specialist ask?

If you have the results of any previous tests, you should take them with you. You may also have been sent a questionnaire to fill in that provides details of your medical history and background. The consultant will usually go over this during your first appointment and ask you and your partner some supplementary questions concerning your personal details and information about your relationship. There will also be questions on your general health, and whether you have any sexual problems. The consultant may also ask you about both your expectations of the treatment and what support you have access to.

Why do I have to answer so many personal questions when seeking fertility treatment?

All clinics offering assisted conception are bound by law (under the 1990 Human Fertilisation & Embryology Act) to provide the HFEA with details of their patients (see p.43) and to take into account the welfare of any child who may be born as a result. This includes both the needs of the child for a father and of any other child or children who may be affected by the birth. In order to establish the welfare of any child you may have as a result of treatment, the clinic will need to ask you a number of searching questions. These will focus on your commitment and future ability to care for a child and to provide for his or her needs. You will also be questioned about any existing or genetically inherited health problems.

Will my religious faith be taken into account?

If you have religious views, for example on the freezing of embryos or selective termination, make sure that the clinic knows what these are – they should be taken into account when you are offered treatment.

Will the clinic contact my GP or anyone else to ask about me?

The clinic will contact your GP and others who might be relevant to their enquiries, such as social workers. They will want to ensure that your GP considers there to be no reason why you or your partner should not be offered treatment. If you refuse to consent to this, it will be taken into account when deciding whether to offer treatment.

What information should the clinic give us before we proceed?

All clinics are obliged by law to give you written information detailing the services offered, together with a full explanation of what treatments involve. They should also provide information on costs, live birth rates and details of their complaints procedure. The HFEA's Code of Practice details the information clinics should provide.

Will I be charged for the initial appointment and how long is it likely to last?

If you are an NHS patient, you won't be charged for this appointment. If you are self-funding at an NHS hospital (see p.162) or having private treatment (see p.163), you will be charged. A typical appointment charge for self-funded treatment is £100 and for private treatment £120. Sometimes the initial consultation is included in the overall treatment package.

What tests am I likely to have at this stage?

Fertility tests fall into two main groups:

Basic tests done to determine whether you are able to conceive:

- Ultrasound scan and blood tests to establish whether you are ovulating.
- Semen analysis to check the number and quality of your partner's sperm.
- Laparoscopy, hysteroscopy and/or hysterosalpingogram to determine the health of your fallopian tubes.

More specialised tests if the diagnosis is unclear:

The precise tests performed will depend on the clinic you attend and the specialist you see.

When will tests be performed and in what order?

You may be given a scan on your first visit to the clinic, but the other basic tests should be done soon after. Consultants may vary in which tests they do when, but they must be done before your next appointment in order to provide you and the consultant with information on which to base further decisions about your treatment.

Be as proactive as you can at this stage. Ask your consultant why they have chosen the test they recommend and whether this is the most suitable option. If they go on to recommend a course of treatment, ask how successful they think the treatment will be and how long the process is likely to take.

Who will be tested first, me or my partner?

Tests will usually be carried out simultaneously over the same time period so that the consultant can review the results and see where your precise problems lie.

I've been told I need to be screened for chlamydia. Why?

Chlamydia is a common sexually transmitted infection. In up to 70 per cent of cases the condition is 'silent', causes no symptoms and so doesn't get treated. It is the main cause of PID, which in turn is the major cause of tubal blockage. It also increases the risk of ectopic pregnancy (see p.120) and chronic pelvic pain. Just one episode of PID confers a 10 per cent risk of tubal blockage, increasing to 50 per cent after three episodes. Procedures such as laparoscopy and dye, HSG and various assisted conception techiques can reactivate chlamydia and increase the risk of PID, so it's usually recommended that women are screened for chlamydia and, if necessary, given a course of antibiotics to clear the infection before undergoing investigative tests.

How long will it be before we get the results of any tests?
Tests should be completed without undue delay. A reasonable timescale – unless there are specific reasons why this cannot be done – would be to have all your tests conducted within six to eight weeks of your first consultation. More specialised tests (such as laparoscopy and dye or post-coital test) will usually be done as and when you need them. There can be up to a one-year wait to have these tests, so always ask what timescale you can expect.

What may the tests show and will this be explained to me?
Once the test results are in, the consultant should have a clearer picture of what is causing your infertility and whether the problem lies with you, your partner, or a combination of both. At your next appointment they should explain what the tests have shown and discuss a proposed treatment plan with you. This may be a drug regimen only, or a combination of drugs and treatments (see p.68).

How will the tests be done and what will they show?
The type of tests and the order in which you are given them will depend on the clinic and the consultant in charge of your care. Although some tests follow a logical order, others may be done to give the consultant a clearer idea of what your specific problem might be. Sometimes it is not exactly clear what the problem is until you have undergone a cycle of assisted conception.

ULTRASOUND SCAN
What it is
Sound waves are used to produce an image of your reproductive system which can be viewed on a monitor.

Why it is done

To assess the health of your ovaries and uterus and see how well the ovaries function. It can show if the follicles (egg sacs) are developing and whether you have problems such as fibroids, polycystic ovary syndrome or abnormalities in the lining or structure of the uterus.

When it is done

An initial ultrasound will normally be done between days two and five of your menstrual cycle. A series of ultrasound scans (two to four) done in the first part of the menstrual cycle leading up to menstruation can be used to follow the development of the follicle and check if an egg is developing. This is known as follicle tracking.

How it is done

It can be done by passing the ultrasound probe over the surface of the abdomen. In this case you will need to drink two pints of water an hour before your appointment in order to fill the bladder (distending the abdomen and allowing a clearer image). You may be given a vaginal ultrasound in which a (lubricated) probe is inserted into the vagina. In this case, your bladder will need to be empty.

BLOOD TESTS

What they are

One or more samples of blood are taken to assess your overall health and to measure your hormone levels. These may help to establish whether you are ovulating and if not, why not.

Why they are done

There are various reasons:

- To check for levels of progesterone (ovulation blood test) if you have regular periods.
- To measure levels of LH and FSH. If levels are low, pituitary hormone treatment may be needed. Raised levels may signify PCOS. Very high levels of LH and FSH can indicate premature menopause.
- To measure prolactin, the hormone involved in milk production. If raised, this may sometimes affect ovulation. However, raised levels are common and don't always need treating, so if your menstrual cycle is regular you won't be offered this.
- To measure testosterone. Raised levels can be a sign of certain types of PCOS and (rarely) other diseases of the ovaries or adrenal glands.

- To measure thyroid hormones. These are rarely a cause of
  ovulation failure and tests will only be offered if you have an
  irregular menstrual cycle or symptoms of thyroid disease.

When they are done

The ovulation blood test is done seven days before your next period
is due if you are menstruating regularly. FSH and LH blood tests are
best done during the first week of your menstrual cycle and will
often be taken on the day you have your ultrasound scan.

How they are done

By withdrawing a sample of blood, usually from the inside of your
elbow using a fine syringe.

HYSTEROSALPINGOGRAM (HSG)

What it is

An X-ray procedure that involves passing dye into the uterus and
fallopian tubes in order to check their health.

Why it is done

To check whether the body of the uterus is normal and whether the
fallopian tubes are open and healthy. It can reveal any adhesions,
fibroids or polyps inside the uterus, show if the fallopian tubes are
blocked or kinked, and is very useful for examining the tubal lining.

When it is done

It is carried out during the first half of your menstrual cycle once you
have stopped bleeding and before ovulation has occurred, ensuring
you are not pregnant, as radiation can damage the embryo.

How it is done

Dye is injected through the cervix and a number of X-rays taken. The
whole procedure takes about 20 minutes and is done in the X-ray or
'imaging' department of the hospital.

When might I be offered it?

If your consultant thinks ovulation failure is the most likely cause of
your problem and considers you are at low risk of having tubal
blockage, you may be offered HSG to avoid the need for a more
invasive laparoscopy. If there is evidence of tubal blockage, a
laparoscopy can be done afterwards. However, if the HSG does not
show up any problems, you may be given drugs at this stage to
encourage ovulation (ovulation induction – see p.68). If after six
months you have not ovulated, you may then be given a laparoscopy.

Does it hurt?
Discomfort is usually minimal but you may experience cramping similar to period pains during and, for a short while, after the test.

HYSTEROSCOPY
What it is
A procedure in which a telescope with a camera attached (hysteroscope) is inserted through the cervix into the uterus.
Why it is done
To check for adhesions, fibroids, abnormality of the structure of the uterus or polyps (growths) in the body of the uterus, which may need to be removed.
When it is done
In the early half of your menstrual cycle so that the doctor's view is not obscured by the build-up of the endometrium.
How it is done
A solution of saline is used to distend the cavity to give a clear picture. The findings are normally recorded on videotape, which can be viewed afterwards at your follow-up consultation.
When might I be offered it?
Hysteroscopy is considered by some specialists to be the best way of detecting abnormalities of the uterus.

LAPAROSCOPY AND DYE
What it is
A laparoscopy provides a view of the exterior surfaces of the uterus and fallopian tubes. A laparoscope is inserted through a small incision in the abdominal wall. Coloured dye is injected via the cervix to see if it flows through the fallopian tubes. Fertiloscopy is a new alternative to laparoscopy, combining dye-test, salpingoscopy, hysteroscopy and microsalpingoscopy. It can be used to investigate unexplained fertility and tubal disorders (see www.fertiloscopy.com for more information).
Why it is done
Tubal blockage is found in 12 to 30 per cent of couples with fertility problems. Laparoscopy allows the doctor to check the health of the fallopian tubes and for endometriosis, fibroids, polycystic ovaries, ovarian cysts, and identify any adhesions or abnormalities of the uterine structure.

When it is done

It can be done at any time in the menstrual cycle, provided you are not bleeding heavily. If the operation is to be carried out after the tenth day of your cycle, you will be advised to use prophylactic contraception while waiting for the procedure as an early embryo conceived at this time could possibly be damaged by the procedure.

How it is done

It is usually done as day surgery under local or general anaesthetic, or you may be admitted to hospital overnight. Your abdominal cavity will be inflated with carbon dioxide to separate the organs and allow a good view down the telescope. The laparoscope is inserted into a small incision close to your navel and dye injected through the cervix. The surgeon can trace it as it flows through the uterus and into the fallopian tubes. If these are open and healthy (patent), the dye will run through them. The whole process takes about half an hour.

When might I be offered it?

Most doctors consider laparoscopy the 'gold standard' for checking the health of the fallopian tubes. It is essential if you have risk factors for PID and/or tubal blockage (eg a history of endometriosis or chlamydia). Similarly, if a blood test has shown antibodies to chlamydia, if you have secondary infertility (and thus are more likely to have pelvic disease), if you have been unable to conceive for three years or more or if you are older and have a lower chance of conceiving without the aid of treatment, you will be offered it.

Are there any risks?

Like any surgical procedure, laparoscopy does carry a risk of complications, as does general anaesthesia. If you are in good health, these risks are small. You may, however, feel bloated and uncomfortable for 24 hours afterwards. There is a slim risk of problems, including infection and injury to the bowel or blood vessels. However, when performed by an experienced surgeon, these are minimal and the benefits more than outweigh the risks.

HYSTEROSALPINGO-CONTRAST SONOGRAPHY (HyCoSy)
What it is

A fairly new, non-invasive technique using transvaginal ultrasound to view the fallopian tubes. It can be done in outpatients and does not involve an overnight stay, but it is not yet widely available.

Why it is done

As an alternative to an HSG or laparoscopy to check fallopian tube blockage. If it reveals abnormalities, the consultant can accurately identify if laparoscopy would be beneficial, and can schedule an appropriate operating time (eg to deal with an ovarian cyst) for you.

It sounds like a better alternative; is it?

The test can confirm very early on that your uterus and ovaries appear normal, that you are ovulating and that your tubes are patent. You can then move on rapidly to the next stage of treatment, thus avoiding a possible long waiting list for a laparoscopy. However, it may miss some types of mild adhesions and endometriosis.

When it is done

HyCoSy can be done at a very early stage in the investigation process and can be combined with a baseline ultrasound test of the pelvis.

How it is done

A catheter with a small deflated balloon on the end is inserted into the uterus through the vagina and cervix. The balloon is then inflated so as to keep the catheter in position. Fluid is injected into the uterus through the catheter. An ultrasound probe is inserted into the vagina, allowing the consultant to see the flow of the fluid through the fallopian tubes. The whole procedure takes just 15 minutes and you can usually go home after half an hour.

When might I be offered it?

If your consultant has reason to suspect your tubes may be blocked (eg if you have a history of chlamydia or PID) they may offer you HyCoSy early in the investigation process. Alternatively, some doctors view the procedure as complementary to laparoscopy (see above).

Does it hurt?

Any slight discomfort is usually minimal.

Will my partner have to have any tests?

Firstly the consultant will establish your partner's sperm quality.

SEMEN ANALYSIS (sperm count)

What it is

A sample of semen is taken to check

- how many sperm there are (their number).
- how active they are (their motility).

- the volume of seminal fluid (the fluid in which the sperm are carried). Too little can make it difficult for the sperm to be transported, too much can over-dilute the sperm.
- the normality of the sperm's appearance under a microscope (their morphology).
- whether there are antisperm antibodies. These can cause sperm to 'clump' together so they are unable to reach the egg.

Why it is done

Around seven out of 10 cases of male fertility problems are due to a low sperm count, although this alone is not usually the prime cause of difficulty in conceiving.

When it is done

Your partner will probably be given a number to call to arrange appointments, as usually two or more tests will be done to assess any variations in sperm production. He should abstain from sex or masturbation for three days before the test.

How is it done?

Your partner will need to produce a sperm sample by masturbating into a sterile pot either at home (if you live near enough to the clinic to get the sample there within at least an hour) or at the clinic. It is usual for your partner to feel embarrassed about this or unsure if he will be able to produce a sample. The staff at the clinic are aware of this and will do their best to make things as easy and comfortable as possible.

My partner has already had his semen tested. Why does it need to be done again?

Even if your partner has already had a semen analysis at the GP's surgery, it will be repeated so that a sample can be looked at in more detail. It takes 10 weeks for sperm to fully mature. During this time, they can be affected by illness and other factors such as smoking and drinking. In order to ensure that a different population of sperm is analysed, another sample is generally taken two weeks later. If your partner has been asked to make lifestyle changes or take antibiotics, another test will be taken 12 weeks later to see if the result improves.

What is a post-coital test and am I likely to have one?

A post-coital test (the cervical mucus sperm penetration test, or PCT) is a test carried out on the woman to find out how well sperm can swim through the mucus in the cervix (the neck of the womb). Many clinics now think that this test is not particularly useful in determining a couple's fertility (ie a sperm that is able to swim through the cervical mucus may still be unable to penetrate an egg). In addition, there are now newer 'sperm function' tests that bypass the cervix. Whether you are offered it will reflect your consultant's view on its usefulness. If you are not offered it, you may want to find out why your consultant thinks it is unnecessary and whether they plan to use any other sperm function tests to determine how well the sperm are able to penetrate the egg.

How is the post-coital test done?

The test is done by examining the cervical mucus six to 36 hours after having sex. Because the consistency and quality of cervical mucus changes throughout the menstrual cycle, the test should be done very close to ovulation and a blood test will be done daily in the run up to your expected time of ovulation to make sure the test is done at the right time. For the best results, you and your partner should abstain from sex for around three days before the test.

When the blood tests identify the LH surge that predicts ovulation, you should have sex that night. The next morning you will be asked to come to the hospital and a sample of your cervical mucus will be taken and examined under a microscope to assess the number and motility of your partner's sperm. If there are few or no active sperm, this may be due to abnormal sperm, abnormal mucus or both. If the sperm are inactive, this may be due to anti-sperm antibodies in the semen or the cervical mucus or to some other abnormality of the mucus, such as over-acidity, that may make it 'hostile' to sperm.

If the test was done too early or too late in the menstrual cycle, or if it was done in a cycle when you didn't ovulate, it may have to be repeated.

What is a normal sperm count?

Although semen analysis is often described as sperm count, numbers of sperm alone are not a good indicator of fertility. For this reason the consultant will take into account other aspects of sperm health to come up with an analysis of semen that includes:

- Volume: there should be between two and five millilitres of sperm.
- Numbers: there should be more than 10 million sperm per millilitre.
- Motility: 40 per cent of the sperm should be actively moving.
- Morphology (shape and structure): 60 per cent of the sperm should be normal in appearance.

My partner has been told he has a low sperm count. What does this mean?

In the past a low sperm count (oligospermia) was considered to be less than 40 million per millilitre. It is now known that men with much lower counts (less than 10 million per millilitre) can still fertilise an egg, provided their partner is under 30 and has no fertility problems. It is important to remember that sperm count alone does not determine male fertility. Men with normal sperm counts can be severely subfertile, while others with low counts can have normal fertility.

What can cause low sperm count?

If sperm count is very low (ie fewer than 5 million) and levels of gonadotrophin hormones are raised, this is a sign that the testes are probably beginning to fail. If there is a complete absence of sperm (azoospermia) and levels of gonadotrophins are very high, it is usually a sign the testes have failed. With newer treatments such as ICSI (see p.104) in which a single sperm is used to fertilise an egg, the quantity of sperm is far less important than its quality. However, where testicular failure has begun, the consultant will usually advise starting treatment as soon as possible and perhaps freezing sperm for future use, in case sperm production fails altogether.

Are there any other causes?

Other causes of azoospermia may be absence or blockage of the vas deferens (the tubes along which sperm pass from the testes to the epididymis) or of the epididymis itself (the tube on the surface of the testes where sperm mature before being released at ejaculation) and varicocele (see p.64). Other external factors can affect sperm count (see p.14).

What is low sperm motility and if my partner has it, how can it affect my chances of conception?

Motility is the ability of sperm to actively move forward. If sperm are being produced but their movement is slow, they are not moving in a straight line, or both, they will have difficulty reaching and/or penetrating the egg. In order to increase the chances of conception, 40 per cent of sperm should be actively moving within an hour of ejaculation. Sluggish sperm may also have other abnormalities that make it impossible for them to fertilise an egg.

What is meant by the term 'abnormal sperm'?

The shape and structure of the sperm is even more important than their number or motility in determining the chances of conception. The perfect sperm should have an oval head and a tail seven to 15 times longer than the head. Abnormalities include having a large round head (indicating that the genetic material inside the cell is unravelling early), a small pinpoint head, a tapered head, crooked head, two heads or a kinked and curled tail. Abnormal sperm are unlikely to be able to fertilise an egg.

Is there anything that can be done to improve sperm quality?

If sperm count is between five and 15 million, the consultant may suggest treatments to try to improve its quality. This may include checking for anti-sperm antibodies and identifying infections that may be causing inflammation of the testes. Treating infections with antibiotics helps to reduce the number of toxins produced by white blood cells, part of the immune defence system, which are produced to fight infection. Clues that he may have an infection include a history of prostatitis (inflammation of the prostate), urethritis (infection of the urethra) or epididymitis (infection of the epididymis).

What are anti-sperm antibodies and do they affect men or women?

Anti-sperm antibodies are protein molecules found in the blood and semen in men or cervical mucus in women. They latch onto the surface of the sperm and may hinder its ability to fertilise an egg. They can prevent conception by causing sperm to clump together, by slowing its ability to swim through the cervical mucus or by preventing sperm from binding to and penetrating the egg. They are more commonly found in men but are also found in women. In men, they may develop after a vasectomy, following an injury or infection of the testicles. It is unknown why they develop in women.

When might we be tested for anti-sperm antibodies?

Research suggests that anti-sperm antibodies affect some five to 10 per cent of couples who seek fertility treatment. The prevalence of antibodies jumps dramatically in men who have had surgery on their reproductive tract: nearly 70 per cent of men who have undergone a vasectomy reversal will have antibodies present in their sperm. However, there is no clear consensus as to how they affect fertility and how much their presence affects the chances of conception. For this reason, testing for anti-sperm antibodies is not routinely offered, but is reserved for couples with unexplained infertility.

Is there a treatment for the presence of anti-sperm antibodies?

Suppressing the immune system with corticosteroids may decrease the production of antibodies but can result in serious side-effects, including severe damage to the hipbone. Intrauterine insemination (IUI), with or without the use of fertility drugs, has been used for the treatment of anti-sperm antibodies, as the process bypasses the cervical mucus. However, IVF appears to be the most effective treatment for very high levels of anti-sperm antibodies.

What is a sperm invasion test and when might it be done?

A sperm invasion test may be done if you have had several post-coital tests which are all negative. A sample of semen and cervical mucus are placed next to each other on a glass slide. This is observed in the laboratory under a microscope to see if the sperm swim through the mucus and remain active (motile). If the mucus is hostile to the sperm, the sperm may have difficulty swimming into the mucus and any that do may stop moving.

I've been told I produce mucus hostile to my partner's sperm. What does this mean and what treatment may be needed?

Cervical mucus problems are responsible for three per cent of cases of female infertility. Normally, cervical mucus is thick and sticky and helps prevent bacteria entering the uterus. However, around the time of ovulation, it becomes thin and stretchy so as to help sperm swim up into the uterus. In some women, the mucus doesn't become receptive to sperm in this way and so hinders the sperm from reaching the egg. Some women make antibodies to their partner's sperm (see above). It is possible to bypass hostile mucus using IUI but in severe cases it's probably more successfully treated with IVF.

I've been told I am not ovulating. Why is this and what treatment may be needed?

Ovulatory problems are by far the most common cause of female fertility problems, accounting for 20 per cent of infertility cases. If you have irregular or absent periods, you may have already suspected that you are not ovulating. However, this is usually confirmed by blood tests. Ovulation failure can happen for several reasons and treatment will depend on the cause.

- Polycystic ovary syndrome (PCOS). This is the most common cause of anovulation (failure to ovulate). It results in high LH levels, low FSH levels and higher than usual production of androgen hormones. Because ovulation is not happening, progesterone is no longer produced, although oestrogen levels remain normal. Treatment with clomiphene citrate (Clomid) or other fertility drugs is often successful, as is ovarian drilling (see p.80). IVF is usually recommended if these treatments are not successful. PCOS is also linked with insulin resistance whereby the body makes, but is unable to respond normally to, insulin. Insulin-lowering drugs can be beneficial in lowering testosterone levels and improving cycle regularity and infertility in PCOS, although further research is determining the relative benefit of these agents over existing fertility measures (see p.68 for more information on fertility drugs).

- Overactive pituitary gland causing high levels of the milk-producing hormone prolactin (hyperprolactinaemia). This is usually caused by small benign tumours or microprolactinomas. Symptoms include irregular cycles, a milky discharge from the nipples and sometimes visual disturbances or headaches as occasionally a tumour can expand and cause pressure effects in the brain. Treatment with the drug bromocriptine or cabergoline will usually suppress excessive prolactin and restore ovulation. Very occasionally, surgery is necessary to remove the tumour.

- Premature ovarian failure (POF or premature menopause). If your ovaries run out of eggs before the age of 40, you will be diagnosed as having POF. This condition often runs in families. The only treatment is IVF using donor eggs.

I've been told I have a luteal phase defect. What is this and what treatment may be recommended?

The luteal phase is the second half of the menstrual cycle following ovulation, during which time the developing dominant follicle is transformed into a body called the corpus luteum (literally yellow body). This produces progesterone in order to prepare your uterus for a potential pregnancy (see p.11). In most women, the length of the luteal phase is 14 days. However, some women have a shorter luteal phase, which can result in a drop in progesterone and loss of this support for the fertilised embryo. You will be treated with fertility drugs to regulate your cycle and encourage ovulation.

I've been told my fallopian tubes are blocked. What may have caused this and what treatment may be recommended?

Fallopian tube damage or blockage is responsible for 15 per cent of female infertility cases. The most common cause is infection caused by chlamydia (see p.46). It is also caused by infection after miscarriage or abortion, endometriosis (see below), childbirth, appendicitis, abdominal surgery or, in older women, tubes may simply become 'worn out'. If your tubes are blocked, you may be offered tubal surgery (laparotomy) for which there are various procedures:

- Laparoscopic microsurgery (keyhole surgery). A laparoscopy is performed, the tube is gently opened up and the damaged portion removed or cleared using a laser.
- If the blockage is close to the uterus (proximal fallopian tube obstruction), it can often be opened up by inserting a deflated balloon on the end of a catheter under X-ray guidance, through the uterus and into the tube where it is then gently inflated.
- A similar technique involves placing a catheter into the fallopian tube by hysteroscopy (a fibre-optic telescope which is placed into the uterus through the cervix) in combination with laparoscopy.

Susan Mitchel

We'd just embarked on infertility investigation in 1998 when I discovered I was pregnant. By that stage, we'd been married for nearly four years and the news came as rather a shock. I think we'd given up hope that it would ever happen and I'd convinced myself that, like my mother and both her sisters, I was moving swiftly towards the menopause. I was 32 at the time and I'd already been told that my FSH levels were on the high side. Sadly, when we went along for the 12-week scan, no heartbeat could be detected. The fetus had probably died at just 10 weeks old. I began to think that maybe my eggs really were past their 'sell-by' date. This seemed to be confirmed when another year went past without anything happening at all. By the end of 1999, we'd started infertility treatment. The doctors kept saying that I'd got pregnant before so it wouldn't be long before I was pregnant again. I found this complacency frustrating but it was also dangerous as I really wanted to believe them. The last thing I wanted to do was sign up to lots of invasive treatment if I didn't really need to.

At the time I didn't realise the significance of a high FSH level. Now, however, I know that some clinics will even refuse to treat women whose FSH is higher than normal. The trouble was that I was (and am) still having periods and I thought that only when they stopped or became irregular would the menopause kick in. I've since found out that there's an initial state called the perimenopause, which can last for several years. During this time, your fertility is reduced and your chances of conceiving are growing smaller all the time.

Fertility treatment didn't work for us. Two IVF cycles were cancelled because my ovaries just didn't respond to the drugs, another sign (so we were told) that my ovarian reserve was low. At that point we decided to stop and take stock and find out more about alternative therapy.

I'd never smoked and I'd already stopped drinking but I started to look at our diet and tried to introduce lots more vegetables and eat only organic meat. I joined a 'Well Woman' yoga class and began to get into chanting and strange, upside-down positions. I went to see an acupuncturist who advised me to cut wheat out of my diet and a reflexologist who claimed that it was possible to turn back premature menopause and become fertile again. I was totally persuaded that both these therapists could 'cure' me, but when four or five sessions failed to produce any results, my natural scepticism returned and I gave up.

The only course of treatment I did stick to was hypnotherapy. The practitioner told me she'd treated lots of infertile women, many of them older than me. Her stories of these delighted women returning with their babies I found very compelling and I willingly, though rather nervously, submitted myself to lying on her sofa every few weeks as she talked me down flights of steps and out into beautiful gardens or along seashores. Her theory was that fertility often becomes blocked by mental stress or problems from the past and that only by exploring the subconscious mind can these blockages be removed.

Hypnotherapy didn't make me pregnant but it did go a long way towards making me more relaxed. The headaches I'd been plagued with for years disappeared and I returned to conventional treatment feeling much more able to cope with it.

You may also be offered surgery if you have:

- scar tissue as a result of endometriosis or inflammation.
- blocked tubes or scarring near the uterus.
- been sterilised. This can be reversed by a procedure called tubal reanastomosis, which usually involves a larger abdominal incision being made in the abdominal wall.

What are my chances of getting pregnant after tubal surgery?

This will depend on why your tubes are blocked and how badly they are damaged. If damage is relatively minor and the blockage is close to the uterus, it is often possible to clear it successfully and for conception to occur. However, if a fallopian tube is severly damaged, particularly if the blockage is at the end of the tube, your chances of conception may be relatively low – even if the tube can be surgically re-opened. By contrast, reversal of sterilisation is often successful.

Are there any risks?

The fallopian tube is more than just a canal for sperm, eggs and embryos to pass down. Its delicate inner lining is actively responsible for nourishing and transporting the embryo to the uterus. If you have tubal disease, despite having surgery, this inner lining may be irreparably damaged with the result that it may become reblocked. Even if you do conceive, you will still be vulnerable to an ectopic pregnancy, which would not be viable. It may also be life-threatening (as it would cause fallopian tube rupture) and would have to be terminated. If your fallopian tubes are irreparably damaged, IVF may be more successful and less risky in terms of ectopic pregnancy.

I've been told I have endometriosis. What does this mean and what treatment may be recommended?

Its cause is unknown. One theory is that during menstruation some menstrual tissue backs up through the fallopian tubes, implants in the abdomen and grows. Some experts believe that all women experience some menstrual tissue back-up and that an immune system or hormonal problem in endometriosis sufferers allows this tissue to grow. These fragments (endometrial cysts) respond to the normal hormones of the menstrual cycle and bleed with each period, causing the formation of scar tissue and inflammation.

Another theory suggests that endometrial tissue is distributed from the uterus to other parts of the body through the lymph or blood system. A genetic theory suggests that it may be carried in the genes in certain families or that some families may be predisposed to endometriosis. Another theory suggests that remnants of tissue from when the woman was an embryo may later develop into endometriosis, or that some adult tissues retain the ability they had in the embryo stage to transform reproductive tissue.

The condition can cause infertility in several ways:

- Endometrial cysts may block the fallopian tubes and prevent the egg from passing down the tubes, or may grow in the ovaries and prevent the release of the egg.
- Webs of scar tissue (adhesions) may develop between the uterus, ovaries and fallopian tubes, preventing the egg from passing down the tube.

Treatment may involve tubal surgery, laser treatment or diathermy (heat treatment) to remove adhesions and scar tissue. Drug treatment may be given after surgery to suppress the activity of the ovaries and therefore slow endometrial-tissue growth. Examples of drugs used include oral contraceptives, progestins, danazol and GnRH (gonadotrophin-releasing hormone) agonists. (GnRH agonists are substances that first stimulate the release of gonadotrophins from the pituitary gland but later suppress gonadotrophin release when administered for more than a few weeks.)

I've been told I have hydrosalpinx. What does this mean?

Hydrosalpinx refers to a collection of fluid that develops in the fallopian tubes when they are blocked at the outer end. The inner end leading to the uterus is open, with the result that the fluid leaks into the uterus and interferes with implantation. Research has shown that the likelihood of pregnancy is halved if you have hydrosalpinx.

Should my fallopian tubes be removed before I have IVF?

If you have hydrosalpinx (see above), fluid in the blocked fallopian tubes can leak into the uterus and prevent implantation. The problem can be avoided by removing the fallopian tubes or clipping them to seal them off (tubal ligation) before having IVF treatment. It's a very difficult step to take because it means that you will never be able to conceive naturally. If you are 35 or younger, you may want to attempt one or two treatment cycles with IVF before taking this step. However, bear in mind that if you have hydrosalpinx it is a sign that your tubes are diseased and the chance of conceiving without assisted conception is very small.

I've been told I have fibroids. What does this mean and what treatment may be needed?

Fibroids – non-cancerous tumours of the uterus – are extremely common in the over 30s. Although rarely problematic, they can affect fertility by making the uterine cavity smaller, blocking the fallopian tubes and altering the position of the cervix, so preventing sperm from reaching the uterus. High levels of oestrogen can stimulate their growth; in this case, surgery to remove them may be suggested.

My partner has been told he has a varicocoele. What does this mean and is there any treatment?

This is the term used to describe dilatation and swelling of the veins that drain the testicle. It affects around 15 per cent of all men and 25 per cent of men attending infertility clinics with a low sperm count. There are usually few or no symptoms, although it may cause a bulge above the testicle in the scrotum, or aching and discomfort. It usually affects the left testis and, as a result of blood pooling, can cause high temperatures in the testis. This can lead to a low sperm count. Operative treatment consists of tying sutures around the veins somewhere between the testicle and the lower abdomen. To do this, most urologists favour an operation where they enter the abdomen. This involves an incision in the groin similar in approach to a hernia repair.

A new treatment for varicocele is embolisation. A catheter is inserted into the affected vein and a liquid containing some tiny stainless steel plugs is passed into the vein to block it off. The procedure is relatively common in the US, although less so in the UK. However, the jury is still out on the value of such treatments. In its infertility guidelines, The Royal College of Obstetricians and Gynaecologists states that there is insufficient evidence to recommend treatment of varicocoele in subfertile men or those with few sperm.

When else might my partner be offered surgery?

With the increasing use of ICSI (see p.104), surgical treatment is used much less for male fertility problems. Surgery is most often used to reverse a vasectomy, to clear blockages of the tubes of the testes, epididymis and vas deferens or to treat varicocoele (see p.64).

How successful is surgery in men?

Surgery is only around 20 to 30 per cent successful in unblocking tubes. The biggest problem is that, after the tubes have been sealed (whether deliberately as in a vasectomy or for another reason), little or no sperm is produced anyway. With the advent of techniques such as PESA and TESE (see p.85), this can be overcome.

My partner has no vas deferens and the consultant has advised him to be screened for cystic fibrosis. Why?

Two-thirds of men with no vas deferens are carriers of the gene for cystic fibrosis, an illness that causes sticky fluid to accumulate in the lungs, resulting in chronic lung infections. There is also an inability to absorb fats and other nutrients from food. The gene is recessive, which means that a baby must inherit a double dose – one from each parent – before the disease causes symptoms. If your partner tests positive, you will also be tested. If you are also found to be positive, you'll be recommended to have full genetic counselling and discussion prior to considering fertility treatment.

We've been told that we have unexplained infertility. What does this mean and is there any treatment?

This is the term doctors use to describe couples – almost a third of all who are investigated – in whom the test results come back normal. This doesn't mean that there is no reason for your infertility. In some cases, you may simply be among the small percentage of couples who take longer than average to conceive. However, where unexplained fertility has lasted for longer than three years, the chances of natural conception are only around 1 to 2 per cent per month (30 per cent over the next two years). As a first treatment option, the consultant may suggest using drugs to induce ovulation combined with IUI, increasing your likelihood of pregnancy to 15 per cent per cycle. If it hasn't worked after six cycles, you will usually be advised to try IVF.

Is fertility treatment our only option?

Not always. It will depend on the problem. Some instances of unexplained infertility involve subtle or minor factors that contribute to your difficulties conceiving. It is important that you get a proper diagnosis and ensure that all avenues have been explored – ie a simple blood test to measure your FSH levels can be a useful guide to whether you are approaching early menopause.

What about complementary therapy?

On the subject of complementary therapy, Professor Robert Winston says: 'I have nothing against alternative or complementary therapy. Many of them will make you feel better, more confident, more relaxed. But there is no clinical evidence to show that they work as an effective treatment for infertility.' However, many couples do find alternative treatments helpful, and some may even claim that it helped them to solve their fertility problems. Acupuncture, Chinese and Western herbal and naturopathic medicine all aim to restore hormone or energy imbalances in the body that may lead to fertility problems. Hypnotherapy aims to confront emotional issues that may prevent conception, as well as strengthening the immune system.

Beware any complementary practitioner who claims a 'miracle cure', and it's advisable to make sure that any complementary practitioner you visit is fully qualified and registered with a professional regulatory body. Many GPs now work closely with alternative practitioners and yours may be able to recommend an appropriate therapist. Alternatively, contact one of the professional bodies listed at the back of this guide and ask them to recommend one in your area. When you call the practitioner, ask them if they have experience of treating people with fertility problems. At the first appointment, establish what the treatments will involve, how many you will need and what possible side-effects may be.

What happens after all the tests?

The consultant should discuss the results of your tests with you and explain your options and the treatment plan they recommend. The options fall into three main categories:

- Fertility drugs
- Tubal surgery

- Assisted conception

If you are being seen in an infertility clinic in a general hospital, straightforward treatments such as fertility drugs and tubal surgery may be available there. If your problems are more complex and/or you need assisted conception, you will usually have to be treated in a specialist assisted conception unit (ACU). These are usually based in the larger NHS teaching hospitals or in a private clinic or hospital.

Should I get a second opinion?

If you are unsure about your diagnosis and want to be certain before going ahead with treatment, you may wish to take your test results to another specialist to see if they recommend the same treatment.

Manchester Health Authority's 2000/01 Policy on the Effective Use of Resources states that patients' requests for a 'second opinion' should, in general, be able to be met by referral to a different provider within existing contract arrangements. If you are using the NHS, you will have to wait to see another NHS consultant in the NHS clinic that you are already using or join a long waiting list to see someone at a hospital with which your PCT has a contract.

If you are using a private clinic, you can arrange a consultation with another private consultant quite easily.

What is 'informed consent' and why is it needed?

As with other medical procedures, any infertility clinic has to, by law, have your written consent to treatment. The HFEA produces a series of quite detailed consent forms that address various issues. By signing them, you agree that you have been given information about the procedures that will be carried out, you have understood the information fully and have had time to consider your decision to go ahead. Forms should include space for you to list any procedures you don't want to have unless you have been able to discuss them fully.

Are there any other legal issues?

Infertility clinics are obliged to pass on information such as your name(s), date(s) of birth and some medical details to the HFEA, where it is held on a computerised register. This is kept because any child born as a result of assisted conception has the legal right to know how she or he came into the world.

Drug treatments

There are many types of fertility drugs and they are used in a number of ways. You may be offered drug treatment alone (to stimulate your ovaries to produce more eggs and to help you conceive naturally) or you may be given drugs as part of assisted conception treatment (for example, to regulate your cycle and prepare your uterus for IVF). Ask your consultant why you are being prescribed certain drugs, and make sure you are clear what function they perfom.

What is ovulation induction and when might I be offered it?
Some fertility drugs work in the same way as your body's own hormones to trigger ovulation. Ovulation induction is often the first – and sometimes only – step in treatment. It is a way of stimulating your ovaries to produce eggs. You are likely to be offered ovulation induction if you have infrequent or absent periods (amenorrhoea or oligomenorrhoea) or have been diagnosed with some types of ovulation failure such as PCOS. The treatment is not just used to stimulate failed ovaries, but also to encourage sluggish ovaries to produce more eggs. This will mean that you produce more than one egg each month, thus increasing your chances of conception. If you are under 35 and there is a relatively straightforward reason why you are not ovulating, ovulation induction is often extremely effective.

Can fertility drugs treat all cases of ovulation failure?
If you are failing to ovulate due to extreme weight loss, a change in diet in order to achieve a more normal weight may be all that is needed to restore your cycle – and your fertility. At the other extreme, if your ovaries have failed as a result of premature menopause, fertility drugs cannot restore ovulation because there are no longer any eggs in your ovaries. Other conditions causing ovulation failure may need more complex medical or surgical treatment. These include:
- hypopituitarism (underactivity of the pituitary gland).
- hypogonadotrophic hypogonadism (poorly functioning ovaries caused by inadequate stimulation of the pituitary by the gonadotrophic hormones).

- hyperprolactinaemia (excessive production of milk-stimulating hormone prolactin), caused by benign pituitary tumour.
- polycystic ovary syndrome (PCOS).

Fertility drugs are often less effective as you get older and the eggs in your ovaries age, so if you are over 35 your consultant may suggest going straight onto assisted conception or limiting the number of treatment cycles using fertility drugs.

What drugs will I be given and what are they used for?

Drugs used to restore ovulation fall into several categories. The tables on pages 70–75 describe some of the kinds of drugs that might be used. There are many fertility drugs available, so if one prescribed for you is not listed, ask your doctor what it is and why it is being used.

My consultant has suggested putting me on Tamoxifen rather than Clomid. Why?

Tamoxifen is a hormonal drug that is widely used to treat – and sometimes to prevent – breast cancer. It works in a similar way to Clomid by blocking the action of oestrogen in the body, and seems to be as effective in inducing ovulation. Your consultant may recommend it because it may have fewer side-effects. It also appears to have less effect on the cervical mucus than Clomid. However, it is still not known what the longer-term effects of tamoxifen may be. For women with breast cancer, there is a slightly increased risk of endometrial cancer (cancer of the lining of the womb). There is no data on the potential risk of ovarian cancer in infertile women treated with tamoxifen, although there does not seem to be an increased risk in women with breast cancer. It is difficult to extrapolate this kind of information on the basis of treatments used in women with breast cancer, as many of them will have passed the menopause or will have had chemotherapy (treatment with cancer drugs) that inhibits the function of the ovaries.

Do fertility drugs cause ovarian and breast cancer?

Many fertility drugs have been used with apparent safety for over 30 years. However, like every drug in existence, those used to induce ovulation have side-effects as well as benefits. In recent years there has been growing concern that fertility drugs may raise the risk of ovarian

DRUGS THAT STIMULATE OVULATION

A number of drugs are used in the early part of the menstrual cycle (when the hypothalamus is stimulating the pituitary to release FSH and LH) to enhance the amount of FSH and/or LH the body produces.

Clomiphene citrate (Clomid/Serophene)

What it is

The oldest and probably the most widely used fertility drug, clomiphene citrate acts on the hypothalamus to stimulate the pituitary gland. This in turn makes the ovaries work harder to produce follicles.

How it works

The exact mechanism by which it works still isn't fully understood. The drug blocks the body's own oestrogen and at the same time acts like oestrogen to first stimulate FSH (the follicle-stimulating hormone) and then, as follicles are produced and levels of oestrogen rise, to inhibit it. Clomiphene has been found to be capable of stimulating a 50 per cent increase in the production of FSH. Ovulation usually ensues within five to 10 days after the last tablet is taken and in women with irregular ovulation the drug seems to re-establish a more normal pattern.

When it might be used

To treat straightforward cases of ovulation failure in women under 40. It is less successful after the age of 40, especially when no clear-cut cause can be established for lack of ovulation.

How it is taken

In the form of a tablet by mouth.

When it is administered

Early in the menstrual cycle – usually on day three to five depending on the length of your menstrual cycle. It is taken daily for five days.

Potential side-effects

Menopausal symptoms such as hot flushes, mood swings, depression, nausea, breast tenderness, insomnia, increased urination, heavy periods, fatigue, skin eruptions and weight gain. Seek medical help if you develop blurred vision or other eyesight changes or experience extreme pelvic or abdominal bloating or pain.

Watchpoints

- Because it blocks oestrogen, it is effective only in women whose bodies are actually producing oestrogen but are not ovulating effectively.
- The drug was originally developed as a contraceptive and may thicken cervical mucus, making it hard for sperm to swim through the cervix and into the uterus.
- Some studies show there may be an increased risk of ovarian cancer following 12 or more cycles of clomiphene. For this reason it is recommended that you have no more than 12 cycles of treatment.
- While taking the drug your ovaries should be closely monitored by ultrasound to check how they are responding and to determine the optimum dose for you.

- The doctor may need to adjust the dosage in ensuing treatment cycles, depending on how your ovaries have responded.
- Clomiphene should only be prescribed by a fertility specialist when a full diagnosis has been obtained and it has been confirmed that the problem is ovulatory failure.
- Your GP should not prescribe it unless you and your partner have had a full assessment and tests (see pp.43–67).
- Clomiphene should not be used if you have liver disease or other dysfunction, as a rare side-effect can be liver problems such as jaundice. Nor should it be used if you have ovarian cysts combined with endometriosis: its use can cause further cysts to develop, which can interfere with follicle development.

Gonadotrophins
What they are
A group of drugs that stimulate the ovaries to ripen follicles and assist in sperm production by enhancing levels of FSH and LH. They include both drugs containing FSH or a mixture of FSH and LH, and human chorionic gonadotrophin (hCG). When ovulation is induced with gonadotrophins you have a 15 to 20 per cent chance of conceiving in each cycle and about a 60 per cent chance after six cycles.

Human menopausal gonadotrophins (hMG), also known as menotrophins eg Humegon, Pergonal, Menogon(r), Menopur(r), made from purified extract of the urine of post-menopausal women or synthetic versions of the same.

Drugs containing FSH alone – these are made from human urine (urofollitrophins) eg Metrodin High Purity or genetically engineered versions of follicle-stimulating hormones (follitrophins) eg Gonal-F(r), Puregon(r).

How they work
By stimulating the ovaries to ripen follicles. Following a course of treatment, ovulation is induced with a single injection of human chorionic gonadotrophin hCG (see below).

When they are used
- When treatment with clomiphene or pulsed GnRH (see below) has been unsuccessful in inducing ovulation.
- If your pituitary gland is not producing FSH and LH eg because of previous pituitary surgery.
- As part of the treatment for assisted conception (such as in vitro fertilisation).
- they are also used to treat male infertility when caused by a condition known as hypogonadotrophic hypogonadism, which depletes sperm.

How they are taken
By daily injections usually for about 10 to 15 days. When ovulation is imminent a single injection of another gonadotrophin, hCG (see below), is given to trigger ovulation.

Potential side-effects

Ovarian hyperstimulation (see p.84), increased risk of multiple pregnancy and miscarriage, hypersensitivity reactions, nausea, vomiting, joint pain, fever and skin reactions at the site of the injection. When used to treat male infertility, they may cause swollen breasts, acne and weight gain.

Watchpoints

- Gonadotrophins are extremely effective but they are powerful drugs and must be given under close medical supervision. You will need to attend the fertility clinic every two or three days to check 1) the number and size of follicles measured by ovarian ultrasound, 2) the levels of oestrogen (to show how much is being produced by the follicles) by blood samples.
- The consultant will usually use as low a dose as possible and increase it only if your ovaries are not responding.

The consultant should first rule out infertility caused by adrenal or thyroid disorders, hyperprolactinaemia or tumours of the pituitary or hypothalamus. Gonadotrophins should not be used if you have ovarian cysts (not caused by polycystic ovary syndrome); cancers of the breast, uterus, ovaries, testes or prostate; vaginal bleeding of unknown cause.

Pulsed GnRH (gonadotrophin releasing hormone, also known as luteinising hormone releasing hormone) eg Fertiral

What it is

A drug based on the hormone produced by the hypothalamus that initiates the whole cycle of ovulation.

How it works

GnRH stimulates the pituitary gland to release FSH and LH, which in turn stimulate your ovaries to develop and release eggs. It mimics your body's own natural production of GnRH, which is secreted (in pulses) every 90 minutes. GnRH stimulates a menstrual cycle that is very similar to your natural one and may reduce the risk of overstimulating the ovaries and multiple pregnancy that many other fertility drugs have.

When it might be used

If your hypothalamus is not producing enough GnRH to stimulate your pituitary gland and you are not ovulating. Doctors refer to this as hypothalamic amenorrhoea.

How it is administered

By means of a small battery-operated infusion pump which is worn continuously for two to three weeks. The pump is attached to a fine tube and needle which is inserted under the skin, or less often directly into a vein.

Potential side-effects

Abdominal pain, nausea, headaches, heavy periods.

Watchpoints

- GnRH will not be prescribed if your lack of periods is caused by being underweight and/or an eating disorder, as it can increase the risk of giving birth to a low birthweight baby and of other problems affecting the baby. The specialist will want to delay treatment until you have got back to a normal weight.

- Success rates don't improve if you take the drugs for longer than six months so discuss with your consultant if, after two or three cycles, you have not conceived.

DRUGS THAT TRIGGER OVULATION
Human chorionic gonadotrophin (hCG) eg Choragon(r), Pregnyl(r), Profasi(r)
What it is
Once the ovaries have been encouraged to produce follicles, other drugs are needed to trigger them to release one or more eggs. The drugs used contain the hormone human chorionic gonadotrophin or hCG, produced in the urine of pregnant women.
How it works
The drugs have the same action as the pituitary hormone luteinising hormone, the surge of which triggers ovulation in a natural menstrual cycle and which also encourages sperm development in men.
When it might be used
- In women to trigger ovulation following administration of other gonadotrophins used to ripen eggs, such as menotrophins or follitrophins.
- In men to treat hypogonadism (deficiency of hormones produced by the testes).

When it is given
The drugs are given when the follicle in the ovary is ripe and ready to be ovulated, normally a day after the last dose of menotrophins or follitrophins. Ovulation typically occurs 36 to 40 hours after the drug is taken, although the precise time may vary from one woman to another.
How it is administered
A single injection, after which you are advised to have sex to coincide with ovulation.
Potential side-effects
Headache, fatigue, mood changes, swollen breasts, skin reactions at the site of the injection, lower abdominal tenderness and fluid retention. May also aggravate ovarian hyperstimulation and increase risk of multiple pregnancy. Thrombosis and rupture of existing ovarian cysts are also a possibility, as is swelling (oedema), especially in men treated with the drug.
Watchpoints
- Should not be taken if you have heart or kidney problems, asthma, epilepsy or migraine.
- Before prescribing it, the doctor should check you have no ovarian swelling or cysts, fibroids or undiagnosed vaginal bleeding.

- During treatment you should have a mid-cycle urine test to check for levels of LH, oestrogen levels should be checked and you will need a mid-cycle ultrasound scan to check for follicle development.
- Seek medical help if you develop severe pain or swelling in the lower abdomen.

DRUGS THAT SUPPRESS YOUR NATURAL CYCLE
Gonadotrophin releasing hormone analogues (GnRH-a) such as Goserelin eg Zoladex(r) (AstraZeneca) and Nafarelin, eg Synarel(r) (Pharmacia)

What they are

A group of drugs that inhibit the release of gonadotrophins (LH and FSH).

How they work

They temporarily reduce the natural production of fertility hormones, prevent the pituitary from releasing LH and FSH and so stop the menstrual cycle. This process is called down-regulation. It permits better control of the stimulation cycle, and helps prevent premature ovulation. In addition, these drugs enable the consultant to choose the optimal time for triggering ovulation.

When they might be used

- In assisted conception treatments such as IVF/GIFT, surrogacy and frozen embryo transfer prior to treatment with fertility drugs.
- To treat endometriosis and fibroids.

When they are given

Nasal spray: one spray into one nostril in the morning and one in the other nostril in the evening, beginning on day two, three or four of the menstrual cycle.

Injectable drugs: as a daily or monthly injection to allow for continuous release of the drug throughout the cycle.

How they are administered

By nasal spray or injection.

Potential side-effects

Because the drug induces an artificial menopause, menopausal symptoms such as hot flushes and night sweats, mood swings, vaginal dryness, headache, irritability, changes in breast size, decreased sex drive, acne, sore muscles.

Watchpoints

- Should not be used if you have pituitary problems or a high risk of osteoporosis.
- Should not be used if you are taking the contraceptive Pill or other hormonal contraception.
- Contact the doctor if you experience palpitations, extreme anxiety or depression, shortness of breath or tightness across the chest, numbness or tingling of hands or feet, rash or itching, abdominal pain or swelling.

DRUGS THAT MAINTAIN PREGNANCY
Progesterone eg Crinone(r), Progynova
What it is

A form of the female sex hormone progesterone, which the body produces during the second half of the menstrual cycle to help the uterus nourish a potential pregnancy.

How it works

By enhancing the body's production of progesterone to help thicken the lining of the uterus (endometrium) to receive a possible embryo, to build protein and store glucose to nurture a possible embryo.

When it might be given

Following embryo transfer in assisted conception techniques such as IVF/GIFT.

How it is taken

By injection into the buttock, vaginal suppository, oral pill or gel.

When it is administered

On the day following the administration of hCG or the day of embryo or gamete transfer, usually around day 15, and continued until eight to 16 weeks of pregnancy.

Potential side-effects

Symptoms associated with pregnancy, such as nausea and vomiting, swollen breasts. Soreness or bruising at site of injection.

Watchpoints

*   Should not be given if you have undiagnosed vaginal bleeding or liver problems.

cancer later in life. Most studies do not show a link but a few do. In the light of this, fertility drugs can now only be prescribed by a fertility specialist. Even where studies have shown a link, it is difficult to know whether this is a matter of simple cause and effect. Some suggest, for example, that women with unexplained infertility have higher rates of ovarian and uterine cancer than other women – whether or not they have taken fertility drugs. A recent study by the London School of Hygiene and Tropical Medicine looked at the incidence of cancer in 5556 women who attended the Hallam Medical Centre, a large infertility clinic in London, between 1975 and 1989. The researchers found the incidence of breast, uterine and ovarian cancers in the women was no greater than expected for the general population.

Further research is clearly needed to establish whether fertility drugs boost the risk of ovarian or breast cancers and to identify which drugs are most likely to do so. Research is also needed to determine at what doses and for how long drugs have to be taken before they increase the risk, and whether some women are at greater risk than others. These have to be weighed against the benefits of using fertility drugs. The Royal College of Obstetricians and Gynaecologists currently recommends that the most widely used fertility drug, Clomid, should be used for no more than six to12 cycles. This is the point at which the likelihood of achieving a successful pregnancy appears to be balanced against any potential risk of ovarian cancer. If you are worried, you should discuss the issue with your consultant, who should be able to tell you about the latest thinking and research.

Does ovulation induction increase my likelihood of multiple pregnancy?

It can do. For example, in one study where women took the two most commonly used fertility drugs, 52 per cent of women taking Clomid and 33 per cent taking gonadotrophins had a multiple pregnancy. The risk appears to be particularly high for women with PCOS treated with gonadotrophins. If you are offered fertility drugs, you may want to discuss your likelihood of multiple pregnancy with your specialist. The risk of multiple pregnancy may be reduced by stepping up drug dosage gradually to find the minimum dose needed to stimulate your ovaries.

Will suppressing and stimulating ovulation bring on an earlier menopause?

There is no evidence that suggests this. The age of menopause is largely genetically programmed and modified by environmental factors such as exposure to radiation, smoking and surgery, that affect the amount of ovarian tissue and/or blood flow to the ovary.

Why are certain drugs needed at certain times?

The natural menstrual cycle is a finely balanced process involving the precise co-ordination of a number of different hormones. Certain drugs must be taken at specific times to mimic your natural cycle and enhance chances of conception (see above). The tables on pages 78–79 explain when each fertility medication is typically administered and why. Use them as a reference but bear in mind that the precise timing of your treatment cycles may vary from this.

How are the drugs administered?

Depending on the drugs, they may be taken by mouth (orally), administered by injection, by infusion pump, as a nasal spray or as a suppository or gel. There are many ways they can be injected: using a traditional hypodermic needle, using a very fine small syringe, using a pen needle, 'gun' or other device to make injecting easier.

I hate injections. Are there any alternatives?

Many people dislike the idea of injections and in some cases there may be an alternative way to take the fertility drugs, such as a nasal spray. Unfortunately, injection is often the best method of getting some drugs into your bloodstream. If you use a syringe with a fine needle, a pen needle or one of the newer methods of administration, you will probably find that injecting is virtually painless.

Can I inject them at home myself?

Most clinics will encourage you to inject the drugs at home as this is more convenient than visiting the clinic daily. The infertility nurse will usually demonstrate how to do this when you are first prescribed the drugs. If you are buying drugs from one of the Home Care services (see p.164) there may be a helpline manned by a specialist nurse who can talk you through your first injection. If you are really

GROUP A

The following medications are administered early in the cycle when the hypothalamus is stimulating the pituitary gland to release FSH and LH. These medications enhance the amount of FSH and/or LH present.

Clomiphene citrate
Clomid®
Milophene®
Serophene®

- Stimulates the hypothalamus to secrete more FSH and LH.
- Taken early in the cycle, usually beginning on cycle day 3 to 5 and continued for five days.

Menotropins
Humegon™
Pergonal®
Repronex™

- A preparation containing LH and FSH.
- It is injected early in the cycle, usually starting around cycle day 5, and continued for approximately seven to 10 days of the cycle.

Urofollitrophins
Fertinex™
Follitrophin beta
Follistim®
Follitrophin alpha
Gonal-F

- Urofollitrophins are preparations containing FSH which have been extracted from the urine of post-menopausal women.
- Follitrophin alpha and beta are synthetic preparations containing FSH.
- They are injected early in the cycle, around day 2 or 3, and continued for approximately six to 10 days.

GROUP B

The following medications are administered in the middle of the cycle when the 'LH surge' is to occur.

Human chorionic gonadotrophin (hCG)
APL®
Profasi®
Choron®
Pregnyl®

- Produces the 'LH surge'.
- It is administered when the follicle in the ovary is mature and prepared for ovulation, usually one day following the last dose of menotrophins or follitrophins.
- Ovulation occurs approximately 36 hours after injection (However, this time may vary for every patient).

GROUP C

The following medications are administered to inhibit the action of GnRH, therefore stopping the release of FSH and LH.

Leuprolide acetate
Lupron®
Goserelin
Zoladex®

- Administered daily, starting around day 21 of the cycle preceding an in vitro fertilisation (IVF) treatment cycle (see below). In certain situations, however, Lupron may be started on the first day of your cycle instead of the preceding cycle (first day of menstrual flow).
- May be given as a monthly injection for endometriosis; this allows for a continuous release of medication throughout the month.

Nafarelin acetate
Synarel®

- A nasal spray preparation.
- Administration begins between cycle day 2 to 4 and continues for approximately six months – indicated for endometriosis.

GROUP D

The following medication is given during the second half of a treatment cycle in order to maintain a pregnancy.

Progesterone
-Crinone®
-Progesterone in Oil injection
-Progesterone intravaginal suppositories
-Progesterone troches
-Prometrium®

- Typically, injectable or intravaginal forms of progesterone are used.
- Administration begins between the day following HCG administration (typically cycle day 15) and continues until a negative pregnancy test or around the 10th week of pregnancy.

GROUP E

The following medication is used to block an early or premature release of LH prior to ovulation so that the specialist can control the timing of ovulation.

Ganirelix acetate
Antagon™

- Used in combination with menotrophins or FSH preparations starting around cycle day 7 or 8.
- This medication is used as part of an IVF treatment regimen.

**Adapted from Stadtlanders Disease Management Division
University of Pittsburgh School of Pharmacy**

squeamish about injecting yourself, you might be able to arrange for the practice nurse to give them at your GP's surgery.

Getting the best from fertility drugs

- Understand exactly why, how and when the drugs are to be taken. If in doubt, check with your consultant or infertility nurse.
- When taking medications daily, it is best to take them at the same time each day to ensure your hormonal levels remain steady.
- Make sure you keep all appointments and attend for any checks designed to measure how your body is responding to treatment.
- If you develop any problems or side-effects, tell your consultant or fertility nurse. Adjusting the dose or changing brands may help.
- Do not ignore symptoms such as rash, swelling, rapid heart rate or shortness of breath – you may be having an allergic reaction.

Does ovulation induction always involve taking fertility drugs?

Ovulation can also be induced by a technique known as ovarian drilling. Used to treat infertility caused by PCOS, the procedure may be done either using a fine hot diathermy probe or a laser under a general anaesthetic. A needle is inserted into the deepest part of the ovary during a laparoscopy. Several holes are made on the surface of the ovary which corrects the abnormal hormone balance found in PCOS. Research suggests that the treatment is as effective in women with PCOS as the use of gonadotrophins. It avoids the increased risk of over-stimulated ovaries that PCOS sufferers are prone to and may help ovarian response to subsequent drug treatment. However, it is a specialised technique and in inexperienced hands can damage other structures in the pelvic area, so it is essential that it is carried out by a doctor trained and experienced in laparoscopic surgery.

Will my partner need to take fertility drugs?

Now that ICSI is such a successful treatment (see p.104), treating male infertility with drugs is not that common. Infertile men with low levels of gonadotrophins can be treated by hCG (see p.73). Hormonal drugs may be used for high prolactin levels due to a pituitary tumour. For poor sperm count, anti-oestrogen drugs can increase levels of FSH and LH and may stimulate testosterone (needed for the formation of sperm). However, none of these treatments is as reliable as ICSI.

Assisted conception

The term 'assisted conception' refers to a range of different techniques such as in vitro fertilisation (IVF) and other related treatments, in which doctors intervene in the process of conception in order to help you become pregnant. The terms assisted reproduction (AR) or assisted reproductive technology (ART) are sometimes used instead.

Each fertility patient is unique, and your treatment may not necessarily follow the same trajectory as someone else's. In order to understand certain procedures, however, it is important to grasp the processes involved in ovulation induction, superovulation and egg collection (whether this is your own or a donor egg) and sperm preparation (whether this is your partner's or donor sperm). These are outlined in the following pages.

What are the different assisted conception techniques?
It can be confusing to be faced with all the jargon and initials used to describe assisted conception. However, there are fundamentally five different techniques:

- Intra-uterine insemination (IUI), also known as artificial insemination (AI), in which sperm are injected high into the uterus. The sperm used may be that of your partner or a donor. If your partner's sperm is used, you may hear it referred to as AIH (artificial insemination by husband) and if donor sperm is used, IUI-D or donor insemination (DI).
- In vitro fertilisation (IVF) in which eggs are fertilised outside the body and replaced into the uterus at the pre-embryo or zygote stage.
- Gamete intra-fallopian transfer (GIFT) and zygote intra-fallopian transfer (ZIFT), in which eggs and sperm (GIFT) or very early pre-embryos or zygotes (ZIFT) are transferred into the fallopian tubes.
- Micro-assisted fertilisation (MAF). These techniques include intra-cytoplasmic sperm injection (ICSI) in which a single sperm is injected into the egg and sub-zonal insemination (SUZI) in which several individual sperm are injected through the external layer of cells, the zona, surrounding the egg.

- Egg or sperm donation in which eggs or sperm collected from a donor are used. The eggs and sperm or embryo can be transferred to the donor recipient by GIFT or IVF. Donor sperm is always frozen to allow for HIV testing and retesting. Fresh eggs are always used because freezing techniques are still experimental.

You'll find more details of each of these techniques on pages 88–105.

When might we be offered assisted conception?

The precise point at which you will be offered assisted conception will depend on the cause of your problems. If your problem is straight-forward, you will usually be offered simpler treatments such as drugs and/or surgery first. If your fallopian tubes are completely blocked, or if you do not respond to treatment with fertility drugs alone, assisted conception may be offered sooner rather than later.

How can we decide whether it is right for us?

Your choice will depend on weighing up your likelihood of achieving a pregnancy using assisted conception against your chances of conceiving using more straightforward treatments. This isn't always an easy calculation – even for experts – and in many cases there is no one right answer. It is important to recognise the benefits and limitations of assisted conception, so arm yourself with as much information as possible including how a treatment may help you and your partner and your particular problems.

How will the consultant decide what kind of assisted conception is most suitable for us?

This will depend on the underlying cause of your fertility problems and how you have responded to any previous treatment. For example, if the problem lies with your partner's sperm, the doctor is likely to suggest ICSI rather than straightforward IVF.

If I need assisted conception, will I have to change hospitals?

It depends where you have been treated so far. Some general hospital infertility units may offer IVF. However, to access the full range of treatment options, you will usually have to go to a specialised high-tech assisted conception unit (ACU) based either in a large teaching hospital or a private clinic.

What should we ask the consultant about assisted conception?

- Why are you recommending this particular treatment at this particular time?
- How much will this treatment increase my chance of conceiving?
- What is the likelihood of me conceiving without this treatment?
- What exactly does the treatment you are proposing involve?
- What are the short-term side-effects or risks?
- Are there any long-term side-effects or risks?
- At what point might you consider that the side-effects or risks of this treatment outweigh the potential benefits?
- Where will the treatment be done?
- How long will treatment take?
- How often will I have to attend the clinic?
- What changes might I have to make in my life while I am undergoing treatment?
- What tests will be performed to see if the treatment is working?
- What will these involve? How am I likely to feel?
- How many treatments do you recommend in order to give me the optimum chance of conceiving?
- Will we be able to store embryos/eggs/sperm for future use?
- Are there any alternatives to this treatment?
- If the treatment is unsuccessful, what are our options?
- How much will the treatment cost? Does this include the cost of drugs and tests that are part of the treatment?
- Will I see a consultant regularly?
- Do you have any information sheets about treatment?
- When do we have to decide whether to go ahead?
- Can you put us in touch with other couples who have had the same treatment?

What is ovulation induction and might I need it?

Also known as superovulation, this is a drug treatment which involves stimulating the ovary to produce two or three eggs, and is usually combined with IUI (see p.88). It is also the first stage of IVF where higher doses of drugs are used to get even more eggs.

Ovulation induction is usually recommended as a first line of treatment for women with healthy fallopian tubes who have partners with a normal sperm count. You will be asked to take the drug clomiphene (Clomid) for five days between days two and six of your menstrual cycle. Your ovaries will be scanned by ultrasound to see how they are responding, and how well your follicles are developing. If you don't respond to Clomid, you may be asked to take injectable drugs, gonadotrophins (see p.71), which are more potent, requiring ultrasound monitoring to check whether more than one follicle is developing (which increases the risk of multiple pregnancy).

What is my follicle count and why is it important?

A count of the number of visible developing follicles (known medically as antral follicles) on vaginal ultrasound is a good predictor of the number of mature follicles that can be stimulated by superovulation. The number of antral follicles is also thought to reflect the relative number of dormant follicles remaining in each ovary. If few are visible, this suggests there are fewer eggs left in your ovaries and these may be poorer in quality, so you are less likely to get pregnant and the consultant is more likely to cancel the treatment cycle. If you have average (or high) numbers of antral follicles, you have a higher chance of getting pregnant. If you fall between these two extremes, it is more difficult to predict the outcome.

What is ovarian hyperstimulation syndrome (OHSS)?

This is a serious complication in which the ovaries become enlarged with fluid-filled cysts. Fluid accumulates in the abdomen, thorax and the sac surrounding the heart. If not diagnosed and treated, it can lead to blood clots in arteries or veins and the risk of heart attack, stroke or amputation. OHSS is more likely to happen if your ovaries have responded especially well to stimulation with fertility drugs. It is also more common in women with polycystic ovary syndrome (PCOS). To minimise the danger of OHSS, the doctor should try to prescribe the lowest dose of drugs needed to produce adequate eggs and will monitor your response carefully. Draining the follicles of fluid at the time of egg collection also helps to reduce the risk.

Symptoms include lower abdominal discomfort, bloating, nausea and vomiting, weakness, faintness and shortness of breath (especially when you are lying down), reduced urine production and in severe cases there may be abdominal pain and the abdomen may be grossly swollen.

If you experience any of these symptoms, it is essential that you seek medical help without delay. If you are being treated in an NHS fertility unit, you should call the unit and report your symptoms. If you are being treated privately, you should call the clinic to tell them but you will usually need to go to your nearest casualty unit and be admitted under the NHS.

A recent study, published in *Human Reproduction*, suggests that one in 20 women given extra hormones to stimulate egg production may suffer from OHSS and recommends natural cycle IVF (see p.99) as a risk-free alternative. However, this is not an option for women with irregular menstrual cycles or who are not ovulating at all.

How is sperm collected and prepared?

If your partner is producing sperm for assisted conception, he will be asked to do so at the clinic early on the day your eggs are collected. The sperm are collected in a sample jar containing a culture fluid or sometimes in two sample jars, to allow the doctor to check that there are sufficient healthy, active ones. The semen is then left for a short period before being washed and prepared (or 'optimised') to select the healthiest specimens. The sperm are spun at high speed in a tube containing a special fluid. If you are using donor sperm (see p.123), this will be thawed from frozen, and prepared in the same way.

In what other ways can sperm be retrieved?

PESA (percutaneous epididymal sperm aspiration) Sperm are retrieved (aspirated) by means of a small needle injected into the epididymis under local anaesthetic.

MESA (micro epididymal sperm aspiration) This is one of the techniques used to retrieve sperm from the epididymis, where sperm is stored. It is used for men who produce no sperm (azoospermia) because of a blocked vas deferens. A small incision is made in the scrotum and fluid extracted from the epididymis which is then examined to see if sperm are present.

TESE (testicular sperm extraction) This is performed if no sperm cells are present in the epididymis. A small sample of the testicle will be taken and examined for sperm cells. The technique is especially useful for men who have previously been sterilised and have tried to have this reversed without success.

Debbie Frankll

When I met my husband to be, he already had two children and had had a vasectomy. Luckily, he was able to have a successful reversal. We decided to wait until we were married before we tried for children. However, after several months I still hadn't conceived and I started to worry. After seeing a leaflet in my doctor's surgery, I made an appointment with a private fertility clinic.

The first thing the consultant did was to take a sperm sample from John. Our worst fears were confirmed when we learned that there were no sperm in the sample and that probably the tubes had reclosed. We were devastated as we hadn't been told that the best time to try for a child was immediately following a vasectomy reversal. The consultant recommended that we go for a second reversal, extracting sperm at the same time and trying an IVF cycle in conjunction with it.

I started on my course of treatment and sniffed the drug Buserelin six times a day to suppress my ovarian function. All the hormones made me very uptight and I suffered hot flushes, forgetfulness, bad mood swings and dreadful headaches. John was constantly supportive while I started my 14-day course of oestrogen injections. These at least made me feel more human again, but they were given intramuscularly and were very painful.

When it was time for my egg collection (under sedation) John was admitted at the same time to have his second reversal, during which they retrieved a lot of motile sperm. These were injected into my eggs by a method known as ICSI. The next day we rang the embryologist who told us that the quality of my eggs had not been very good but at least a few had fertilised. Two days later, the embryos were replaced. We held our breath for 16 days, and were devastated to learn that the blood test showed that there was no pregnancy.

We waited four months and started again. This time I tried to stay calmer and tried hypnotherapy, massage, and finally, my consultant recommended a Chinese herbalist who gave me herbs and acupuncture. The herbs tasted foul (thought to redress imbalances in the body) but the acupuncture was very relaxing (thought to stimulate the flow of energy to the reproductive organs to regulate them). I also joined the support group at the clinic where I found the team very calm and informative.

This time I felt hopeful and out of nine oocytes collected, seven were suitable for ICSI using John's frozen sperm. Three fertilised and all were transferred. Sixteen days later (November 5) my blood test proved positive. We sobbed and told everyone. My scan showed a very strong heartbeat in one embryo and we had the best Christmas ever.

On New Year's Eve I started to bleed. A scan showed that there was no heartbeat. Ten days later, at 10 weeks pregnant, I had a D&C. Our grief was enormous and I couldn't believe that this was happening to us. I was very depressed. Life became very strained for John and I and the only thing that kept me going was knowing that I could get pregnant.

Three months later we tried again. My consultant upped my drug dosages. I kept on with the Chinese herbs and acupuncture. The scans showed several oocytes developing with one always in the lead and bigger than the rest. The twice-weekly blood tests showed good hormone levels. When I went for my egg retrieval there were 14 good quality oocytes and 10 had fertilised when we rang the next day.

I had more acupuncture before the embryos were transferred. Sixteen days later we had a positive pregnancy test. Our scan showed us one embryo. Amazingly, I had a trouble-free pregnancy and after a long labour and emergency Caesarean, our son Jack was born.

FROSTESE (frozen testicular tissue extraction) A piece of the testicle is removed (as in TESE) and frozen. Sperm survives better in testicular tissue than in semen. If fresh sperm is need for a particular treatment, repeated sperm extraction has to be done on the same day as egg collection in order to ensure the sperm is fresh. FROSTESE avoids the need for this and bypasses the risk of post-extraction infection and complications such as bleeding. The samples are frozen and thawed and used in IVF/ICSI.

Does sperm retrieval hurt?

Your partner will usually experience a small amount of bruising and tenderness for a day or so afterwards, but will be back to normal within two or three days. Healing usually takes 10 days to two weeks.

IUI (INTRA-UTERINE INSEMINATION)

IUI involves placing a sample of prepared sperm directly into the uterus via the cervix. The sperm can either be that of your partner or a donor. IUI raises your chance of conceiving by increasing the likelihood of eggs and sperm meeting in the fallopian tubes. Provided your fallopian tubes are healthy and unblocked, with no evidence of endometriosis, the technique can be a useful way to give nature a helping hand. The technique may be used with eggs induced by fertility drugs or with naturally ovulated eggs.

It may be used:

- if you have been diagnosed with unexplained infertility – provided there are no problems with your ovaries and fallopian tubes.
- if your partner has a low sperm count or low motility – provided sperm are normal.
- if you are producing cervical mucus that is hostile to sperm.
- if you or your partner are producing sperm antibodies.
- in the rare instances where sex is impossible and sperm cannot be ejaculated into the vagina.

How is it done?

The procedure is usually performed between day 12 and day 15 of your menstrual cycle to coincide with ovulation. Your follicles will be tracked by ultrasound scan, and once the lead follicle is 18mm in size, you will be given an injection of HCG to mature and release the egg. As this injection takes 36 – 40 hours to work, insemination is timed to coincide with the moment the egg is released into the fallopian tube. The sperm is first washed and prepared (or 'optimised') to select the healthiest specimens. The resulting sperm, together with a small amount of culture fluid, is placed in a catheter (a long, soft, narrow plastic tube). The doctor will insert a speculum into your vagina to keep the vaginal walls apart and to allow him to view your cervix. The catheter is inserted through your cervix to the top end of your uterus where the sperm is released. The tube is then carefully withdrawn and you will be told to rest for a few minutes to allow the cervical mucus to seal off the cervix. After this, you can go home. The procedure is quick and painless and there is no need to take time off work or limit your activities during a treatment cycle.

Is this the same as artificial insemination?
No, with artificial insemination (otherwise known as intracervical insemination) fresh sperm is placed directly into the cervix rather than the uterus, using a syringe and a long, narrow tube called a cannula. However, this technique is hardly ever used.

IN VITRO FERTILISATION (IVF)
Sometimes known as the test-tube technique, there are five key steps to IVF. Ovulation is induced and eggs collected. Sperm is collected and then mixed with the eggs in the optimum conditions for fertilisation and early embryo growth. After this, the resulting embryos are transferred into the uterus. The idea behind IVF is that the chances of pregnancy are increased if more than one egg is obtained, so the aim is to collect eight-12 mature eggs. At the beginning of each cycle, each ovary has a pool of over 20 immature eggs ready to be stimulated and to grow. The drugs used in IVF override the natural hormonal signals which select only one egg to mature and be released. By using a higher dose of the hormone FSH from day two or three of the cycle, several eggs are allowed to grow and mature in each ovary. The growth of the eggs is monitored using ultrasound scans which measure the size and number of follicles. When two or three follicles have reached 18mm in size, the eggs inside the follicles are ready to be collected (see below).

When might it be recommended?

- If your fallopian tubes are blocked or damaged.
- If you are producing antibodies to your partner's sperm.
- If you have hormonal problems.
- If your infertility is linked to endometriosis.
- If your partner has minor problems with fertility.
- If your infertility is unexplained.
- If other techniques, such as IUI, have failed.

How effective is it?

According to the latest data available from the HFEA, the average live birth rate for each treatment cycle is around 19.5 per cent using fresh embryos, and about 13.4 per cent using frozen embryos. It is important to recognise that IVF is not effective for everyone and to an extent your chances of conceiving successfully will depend on the experience and skill of the staff at the clinic. Other factors include:

- your age: IVF is less successful in women over 38 and its effectiveness declines further after 40.
- how long you have had fertility problems and how many you have: the longer you have been infertile and the more problems you have (especially if your partner is also infertile), the lower your chances of conception with IVF treatment.
- The number of attempts at IVF you have: your chance of conceiving is greatest in the first treatment cycle and declines with each subsequent attempt. However, because a few more women conceive with each cycle, the cumulative pregnancy rate (or CPR) continues to increase up to around the sixth cycle where it peaks. After the sixth treatment cycle the CPR declines, especially in women over 40.
- Whether you have primary infertility or secondary infertility: women with secondary infertility are more likely to conceive using IVF than those with primary infertility.

Why are IVF failure rates so high?

They aren't. In fact, the overall success rates of IVF are on average equal to those of women who conceive naturally – around 20 to 30 per cent each cycle – and sometimes better. The chances of continuing the pregnancy and going on to give birth to a live baby are slightly less because many pregnancies are miscarried at an early stage, but this happens in natural cycles too. It is worth bearing in mind that the chances of success increase with each cycle of treatment so that after four cycles your 'cumulative' likelihood of becoming pregnant will be 50 per cent or higher. On the other hand, because fertility decreases with age your chances of successfully conceiving with IVF decreases as you get older. By your early 40s your chance of success is no more than 5 per cent and by 45 virtually nil.

Is IVF the fastest way to conceive?

Improvements in techniques mean that some IVF clinics give couples a higher chance than they would otherwise have naturally. Some clinics in the UK quote a conception rate of 40 per cent per treatment cycle – compared with 20 to 25 for natural conception. Having said that, IVF is complicated, emotionally taxing and expensive and most couples wouldn't choose to use it in preference to conventional conception unless they had a problem.

Can the type of drugs I am prescribed make a difference to my likelihood of getting pregnant using IVF?

There are slight, but nonetheless significant, differences in the likelihood of conceiving using different types of drugs. For this reason the consultant will take a number of factors into account before deciding which drugs are most likely to produce the best result for you. You should ask the consultant why they have chosen the particular combination of drugs they plan to prescribe. They will be taking the following into account:

- The pregnancy rates achieved by taking the drug based on published trials.
- How your consultant thinks your ovaries will respond based on your FSH levels, your age and your previous reponse to any treatment.
- If there is a risk of OHSS (eg if your infertility is caused by PCOS).
- How the drug is administered and how acceptable this is to you. The most recent FSH preparations (see p.72), for example, are now given by injection under the skin, rather than by a deeper – and more painful – injection into a muscle.

How does IVF work?

IVF uses gonadotrophins (see p.71) to coax your ovaries into producing more than the usual number of mature eggs. The more eggs there are, the greater the chances of success using IVF. The sequence of events for superovulation is as follows:

- Your menstrual cycle is suppressed with GnRH-a. The drug is taken in the form of nasal spray, daily or monthly injection from around seven to 10 days before your expected period in the cycle before IVF is planned.
- You will be given injections of hMG or recombinant gonadotrophins (produced by biotechnology). You will need a daily injection to help ripen several follicles to maturity.
- While you are taking drugs, your follicles will be monitored by a system called 'follicle tracking'. The follicles' development is monitored by ultrasound and you may also have to provide blood samples to check your oestrogen levels. In a natural cycle this would stimulate the ovary to produce a single follicle, but as the normal activity of the pituitary has been suppressed, the ovaries can be stimulated to develop more follicles to maturity.
- When the follicles are the right size (they need to be at least 18mm), a single injection of hCG is given to finish ripening the eggs and to trigger ovulation.
- As your own hormones have been suppressed, you will need one or two lower-dose injections of hCG, or progesterone treatment to create a suitable environment for embryo implantation.

How and when are eggs collected?

Your eggs are collected when your follicles are the right size and ready to be ovulated. In order to ensure that the eggs are mature but not yet ovulated and lost, egg collection must take place before the follicles rupture and release the eggs – 36 to 40 hours after the hCG injection. Timing is of the essence as, if egg retrieval occurs too early or too late, the eggs will not develop properly or may be released from the ovary and lost.

Egg collection normally takes 20 to 40 minutes. You will normally be sedated to help you relax, although very occasionally it may be done under general anaesthetic using laparoscopy, although this is more usual if you are having GIFT (see p.102).

Each ripe egg, together with the fluid surrounding it, is retrieved via the vagina using a needle attached to a suction pump under ultrasound guidance. The needle is inserted in the ovarian follicles and gentle suction applied to retrieve the egg, which is then placed in a test tube. This is called 'follicular aspiration'. As each follicle is drained, the test tube containing the fluid and the egg is passed to an embryologist who looks at it under a microscope and transfers it to a shallow glass dish containing a nutrient-rich culture fluid. This is then stored in an incubator.

Will there be any side-effects or complications?

Immediately after egg collection you may feel drowsy from the sedative or anaesthetic. The most common side-effect is a feeling of soreness in your ovaries and abdomen and bloating of the abdomen. You may also experience a little vaginal bleeding. This should be light and not last for more than a couple of days. If you experience heavy or persistent bleeding, contact the clinic. There is a potential risk of infection caused by normal bacteria that inhabit the vagina. The doctor will try to minimise this risk by cleansing the vagina with an antiseptic fluid before retrieving the egg and you may also be given prophylactic (preventative) antibiotics.

How are the eggs fertilised?

Four to 6 hours after your eggs have been retrieved, your partner's or donor's sperm will be added to the eggs. If your partner is providing sperm, he will be asked to do so early on in the day, either at the clinic or at home if you live less than an hour away. After overnight incubation, the eggs are viewed under a microscope to see if any have fertilised. If so, the fertilised eggs (zygotes) will be transferred to a fresh culture fluid and returned to the incubator for a further 24 to 48 hours. If they have not fertilised, they may be re-inseminated or ICSI may be performed (see below). If fertilisation still does not occur, the rest of the treatment cycle will be cancelled (see p.99).

What does the embryologist do?

Embryologists are experts in the formation, early growth and development of living organisms. Clinical embryologists work in fertility clinics with human embryos and are involved in research and laboratory investigation of various aspects of assisted conception techniques. These include egg collection, checking your fertility level, eggs, sperm and any embryos that have been fertilised, analysing the quality of embryos and choosing which ones should be transferred and/or frozen.

When will embryo transfer take place and how is it done?

You will be told to phone the clinic the day after your eggs have been collected to see if any have fertilised. Occasionally, your partner may be asked to supply another sample of semen to re-inseminate the eggs. If the eggs have fertilised, you'll be asked to come into the clinic for embryo transfer – usually two or three days after egg collection. The embryos are transferred to your uterus together with a tiny drop of the culture fluid. A speculum is used to open the vagina and enable the doctor to view the cervix and a small tube or catheter is used to insert the embryo(s) into the top part of your uterus. The catheter is then withdrawn and checked under a microscope to make sure that the embryo(s) have been successfully deposited and after a short rest you'll be able to get dressed and go home. Embryo transfer is usually virtually painless, although you may experience mild cramps rather like period pains.

Can I ask for more than three embryos to be transferred and will this increase my chances of success?

In the UK this is not possible. The most recent HFEA ruling advises that in most cases only two embryos should be replaced, and no more than three, to avoid increased risk of multiple pregnancy and birth with all its potential complications. In some situations – for example if you are between 35 and 40 and have had three or more unsuccessful attempts at IVF – the consultant may suggest replacing three embryos to increase your chances of conceiving. Elsewhere, for example in some clinics in the US, where there is less regulation, three or more embryos are routinely replaced.

What are my chances of having a multiple pregnancy with IVF?

An estimated third of multiple births in the UK today are a result of assisted conception. The precise likelihood depends on how many embryos are transferred and on you (non-identical twins are more common in younger women undergoing IVF). Around 65 to 75 per cent of pregnancies resulting from assisted conception will produce a single baby, 20 to 30 per cent twins and three to five per cent triplets.

What if I only want one child?

Many doctors prefer to replace two eggs or embryos in order to increase your chance of conception, unless you have a medical problem which would make it unwise for you to have a multiple pregnancy or birth. If you only want one child, you should discuss it with your doctor. It may sometimes be possible to have natural cycle IVF. However, you should be aware that if only one embryo or egg is transferred your odds of conceiving are significantly reduced.

Should I take time off work after an embryo transfer?

In the past, when embryo transfer was done via laparoscopy, women were usually advised to take time off work. Today, embryo transfer is usually done via the vagina and although most specialists will advise you to take it easy for a few days there's no need to take time off, unless the ACU is some distance from your home. If your job is physically strenuous or involves a lot of mental stress and rushing around, you may feel more relaxed if you take three or four days off. If you do decide to take leave, it's important to make it an enjoyable time by doing things that you like and not spend it sitting around worrying about whether you have conceived.

Does having sex after transfer increases the success of IVF ?

Most fertility experts advise couples to avoid sex around the time of embryo transfer. However, research done in Australia published in *New Scientist* found that sex in the days around the transfer improved pregnancy rates by 50 per cent. The researchers surmise that an ingredient in semen may prevent the woman's immune system from rejecting the new embryo. On the downside, most of the extra pregnancies were multiples such as twins and triplets. Until more research is done in the UK, experts remain cautious and point out that there is a small risk of the uterus expelling the transferred embryo after sex.

What does the grading system for embryos mean?

Once your eggs have been fertilised, the embryologist will examine them under a microscope to assess their development. The quality of each embryo is scored on a 3 to 5 point scale with perfect embryos graded 1 or A, depending on the system the laboratory uses. The thickness of the egg's protective shell (zona pellucida) will also be considered. A thick zona pellucida can make it more difficult for an egg to be fertilised. Research has shown that embryos with the highest score have round, symmetrical cells, and result in high conception rates when transferred back to the uterus. It is perfectly normal for the embryonic cells to fragment as they divide. However, those that fragment severely will be small and uneven in shape and when transferred back to the uterus (or frozen for future use) will give you a poorer chance of conception. The better the grade of the embryos, the greater your likelihood of becoming pregnant. If you are having embryos frozen, only those with better grades will be chosen.

What is the significance of the embryo cell division rate?

The rate of cell division or cleavage is another indication of an embryo's potential to implant. Research has shown that early cleavage – that is embryos that have divided into four cells by the second day after egg collection and seven to nine cells by the third – are more likely to implant in the uterus and result in a higher conception rate than those with fewer or more cells at these points.

What is blastocyst transfer and could it help me conceive?

Doctors have discovered that as the embryo continues to divide, its quality decreases. One way to select the better quality embryos is to allow them to carry on dividing in a nourishing culture fluid called a sequential medium. On the fifth day after fertilisation, they are replaced in your uterus, which is what would happen naturally. It has been found that replacing the embryo at this stage – known as the blastocyst stage – increases the likelihood of pregnancy.

Are there any risks?

This technique is still fairly new and, as with any other, the long-term outcome is unknown. There were some early concerns about the possibility of high birth weight and congenital abnormalities.

However, hundreds of children have now been born using the technique and these fears have so far proved unfounded. There have also been reports suggesting an increased risk of identical twins – possibly because of changes in the embryo's outer shell which cause the embryo to split in two. One potential pitfall is that in one in 10 cases no embryos survive to the blastocyst stage.

How can we be sure the eggs, sperm and embryos used for IVF are ours?

Clinics licensed by the HFEA are regularly assessed to ensure labelling and checking procedures conform to regulations. These are designed to ensure that eggs, sperm or embryos don't get mixed up. However, in July 2002, there was a highly publicised case of black twins born to a white couple. Safety procedures must include checking your name and date of birth and that of your partner verbally several times and labelling the dishes containing eggs, sperm and embryos as they are collected. Ask your clinic to explain what checks are in place.

Should I freeze any 'extra' embryos after IVF treatment?

You may have several embryos left over after treatment. Cryo-preservation – freezing and storing your embryos – allows you to use them in future treatment cycles. This removes the need for further superovulation and egg retrieval and reduces the emotional, physical and financial toll. Alternatively, you may decide to donate any unused embryos to other couples with fertility problems, or to research.

Freezing may be recommended

- if you are over 40, as a safeguard against the decline in egg quality and quantity as menopause approaches.
- if you experience severe side-effects such as OHSS as a result of taking fertility drugs.
- if you are to be treated for cancer the treatment may make you infertile.

How are embryos frozen?

A kind of chemical 'antifreeze' is used to 'freeze dry' the embryonic cells. These are then stored in liquid nitrogen under carefully controlled conditions, at a temperature of -196 °C. Stored at this temperature, the embryos do not deteriorate and have the best possible chance of survival when rethawed.

How much does it cost to freeze and store embryos?
Costs vary from centre to centre but a typical charge would be £150 for initial freezing and storage (say for up to two years) and an additional £60 a year thereafter.

How long can frozen embryos be stored?
The HFEA specifies that embryos can only be frozen for five years, after which you can apply for an extension of up to 10 years, and in some circumstances for longer. During the storage period the clinic will review your embryos and keep in touch with you. Make sure you tell the clinic if you move or change address.

What will happen when the time limit expires?
At the end of the specified time period any unused embryos must be disposed of. You should make a note of the storage date so that you know when it expires. The clinic will contact you before this date which will allow you to make plans to use them, or decide if you want to donate them to another infertile couple or for use in research.

What is assisted hatching and could it help me conceive?
One reason why women over 40 can find it harder to conceive is because the outer shell – or zona pellucida – of their eggs becomes harder and thicker. Assisted hatching involves making a hole in the egg's shell, either by laser or chemicals, to help the egg to 'hatch' or break out of its shell. The technique is increasingly offered to women over the age of 40 and women who have had three or more unsuccessful attempts at IVF, despite good quality embryos having being transferred.

Are there any risks?
Like any medical procedure, assisted hatching has risks as well as benefits. These include infection or destruction of the embryo by your own immune cells. There is also a potentially increased risk of conceiving identical twins as a result of the embryo splitting in two, hatching one half through the 'hole' and the other breaking through.

Why might treatment be cancelled?

Assisted conception is a complicated process and things don't always go to plan. In about 15 per cent of cases this will mean that the treatment cycle has to be cancelled.

Reasons a cycle might be cancelled:

Before treatment: if it is discovered that you have an ovarian cyst or polyp which needs treating; because frozen embryos have failed to survive thawing (see above).

During superovulation: if your ovaries have become hyper-stimulated or if your ovaries don't respond to the drugs – ie if too few eggs (less than three) develop. Failure to respond is most likely if you are over 40. You will probably be advised to wait another couple of menstrual cycles to rest your ovaries before trying again.

Before collection: if ovulation occurs too soon (and therefore the eggs are not mature enough to be fertilised).

At collection: if sperm is of too poor quality to fertilise the eggs.

Following collection: if the eggs collected fail to fertilise.

How am I likely to feel if treatment has to be cancelled?

However much you try to be realistic, it's natural for hopes to be raised at the start of a treatment cycle and for them to come crashing down if the cycle has to be cancelled. It is common to experience feelings of depression, anger and guilt. It's important to bear in mind that if a cycle has to be cancelled it does not mean that you are a failure or that you will never get pregnant. The doctor should make an appointment to review your treatment and discuss why it had to be cancelled.

Will we have to pay if a cycle has to be cancelled?

You will usually have to pay a certain proportion, depending on the point at which the treatment had to be cancelled. If you have paid for a full package in advance, you will usually be eligible for a refund for the part of the treatment you didn't have (see p.163).

NATURAL CYCLE IVF

Natural Cycle IVF involves collecting and fertilising a single egg ovulated during a natural menstrual cycle rather than using the more usual superovulation. Ironically, although natural cycle IVF is a newly offered technique, the very first test-tube baby born in the UK, Louise Brown, was a result of a natural cycle. Recent research suggests that women having natural cycle IVF can achieve similar results to drug-stimulated cycles after three to four cycles of treatment – 32 per cent of women gave birth to a baby compared with 34 per cent in the drug-stimulated group.

Pros and cons of natural cycle IVF

Pros

- Avoids the need to take costly fertility drugs and so bypasses short-term but potentially dangerous side-effects such as OHSS, as well as any potential long-term risks.
- Minimises risk of multiple pregnancy and birth.
- Can be done every month because the ovaries are not overstimulated, unlike superovulation where treatment may be spread over months or years to allow the ovaries time to recover.
- Saves on cost. Research has found that in the UK natural treatment cycles could be offered at 23 per cent of the price of superovulation cycles.

Cons

- May reduce chance of pregnancy – especially if you are over 40.
- No spare eggs or embryos for freezing should you want to have future attempts at IVF.

Am I suitable for natural cycle IVF?

You might want to consider natural cycle IVF if you have a fairly regular menstrual cycle and are ovulating normally, your fallopian tubes are blocked (which makes IVF the treatment of choice) or you have unexplained infertility. However, if you are not ovulating, your menstrual cycle is very irregular or you and your partner are having ICSI (see p.104), this treatment is not suitable for you.

Where can I get natural cycle IVF?

A growing number of clinics are offering the procedure and with the HFEA's most recent ruling which says that no more than two embryos should be replaced in the majority of cases, together with concerns about the potential long-term effects of fertility drugs, the technique may well become even more widespread in future.

FROZEN EMBRYO TRANSFER (FET)

If, after an IVF cycle, not all your embryos have been used, these can be frozen and stored for use at a later date. A frozen embryo transfer cycle (FET) is less expensive than repeating IVF as you don't need to go through ovulation induction and egg retrieval. Approximately 75 per cent of frozen embryos survive the thawing process, but this varies depending on how long ago the embryos were frozen.

Are there any risks associated with freezing embryos?

Since the mid-1980s, many babies have been born using frozen embryos with apparent safety. However, the long-term effects of freezing embryos are not known and there is still discussion as to whether it may be harmful. Not all embryos survive the freezing process and some may be damaged as they are stored. Around 65 to 75 per cent of embryos survive the freeze-thaw process. The precise figure depends on the clinic and the types of freezing methods they use. The live birth rate per cycle is lower (around 12–15 per cent) than when fresh embryos are replaced because some embryos lose their quality when they are thawed, but the quality of the embryo bears no relation to the health of any resulting child.

Are there any risks associated with Frozen embryo transfer?

Early research suggested that freezing damaged gene control mechanisms and led to a risk of genetic defects. The latest research suggests that this is not the case. All the babies born using frozen embryos so far have been healthy, although some specialists do still have concerns about the risk of congenital abnormality or other problems that may emerge over time.

What about egg freezing?

The human egg is the largest cell in the body and as such is more easily damaged by freezing (ice crystals may form inside the egg). Until recently, fertilisation rates were still dismally low using frozen eggs in conventional IVF. But recently, greater success has been achieved using ICSI (see p.104) and doctors in some clinics do now offer egg freezing, although it is expensive compared with sperm and embryo freezing.

How successful is it?

The use of frozen eggs is still fairly new and untested and to date only a relatively small number of babies have been born using it. The newness of the technique means that it is more difficult to assess the likelihood of success, although as yet pregnancy rates are lower than with conventional IVF or ICSI. This may improve as more is learned about the process.

Thawing eggs is more expensive than thawing embryos, and the quality of the eggs is crucial to their chances of survival. One London clinic that offers egg freezing in carefully selected cases comments in its literature: 'at best, the survival rate for good quality oocytes [eggs] is 57 per cent. The fertilisation rates for conventional IVF using frozen oocytes (that have survived) is reported to be between 30–50 per cent. The fertilisation rate for ICSI using frozen oocytes (that have survived) ranges from 56–64 per cent. Thus cryo-preservation of oocytes is still considered a low efficiency technique.'

When might I consider egg freezing?

If:

- there is a risk of early menopause as a result of cancer treatment or genetic tendency.
- there is a risk of early menopause as a result of a chromosomal abnormality such as Turner's syndrome. The woman's mother or other female relative may decide to freeze eggs while they are still of reproductive age.
- you and your partner have religious or ethical objections to frozen embryos.
- you intend to delay childbearing until later in life and wish to preserve the better quality eggs produced while you are young.

GAMETE INTRAFALLOPIAN TRANSFER (GIFT) AND ZYGOTE INTRAFALLOPIAN TRANSFER (ZIFT)

What is GIFT and when might I be offered it?

Gamete is the medical term for a sperm or an egg. In GIFT, gametes (ie sperm and eggs) are placed in the fallopian tubes. The basic preparatory procedures are the same as for those used in IVF – ie your ovaries will be stimulated using fertility drugs and the eggs will be retrieved as described on p.92. However, it differs from IVF in that fertilisation occurs inside your body rather than in a dish in the laboratory. Once the eggs have been retrieved, up to three mature ones are selected and mixed with sperm (either your partner's or a donor's) and these are then placed into your fallopian tube. The procedure is performed immediately after egg retrieval. GIFT may be recommended if you have been diagnosed with unexplained infertility, you have problems with cervical mucus (eg hostility to your partner's sperm) or you have mild endometriosis. It is not recommended if you have had an ectopic pregnancy (and perhaps lost one fallopian tube) because there is a risk of having another one.

How is GIFT performed?

Your eggs are more usually retrieved by laparoscopy under general anaesthetic. Once the laparoscope is in place, the surgeon gently lifts the outer end of a fallopian tube and threads a narrow rigid metal tube a short way up the tube through an incision in the abdominal wall. The prepared sperm are mixed with the retrieved eggs in a catheter, which is threaded down the fallopian tube into which the gametes are released, and where hopefully they fertilise.

The advantages of GIFT are that it is usually less expensive than IVF and success rates tend to be higher. However, if it doesn't work, it is more difficult to work out why, as it is impossible to tell whether or not fertilisation took place. Some couples are recommended a 'trial' of IVF in order to establish the ability of the sperm to fertilise the eggs. If fertilisation does occur in vitro, GIFT may be appropriate if future treatment is needed.

What is ZIFT and when might I be offered it?

A zygote (sometimes called a pre-embryo) is the medical term for an egg that has fertilised but not yet divided. ZIFT is similar to IVF in that fertilisation takes place in the laboratory. However, the fertilised eggs are transferred on day one. Up to three zygotes can be transferred at a time to the woman's fallopian tube, the idea being that at day one the embryo would normally be in the fallopian tube rather than the uterus, and that this is the ideal environment for it to develop in.

The main disadvantage is that you will have to undergo two procedures – egg collection and zygote transfer (which involves a laparoscopy under general anaesthetic) – one after the other. Also, there is no opportunity to select the best two embryos to transfer, as at the time the zygotes are transferred it is impossible to tell which of the fertilised eggs is developing most promisingly.

MICRO-ASSISTED FERTILISATION (MAF) PROCEDURES

What is ICSI and when might we be offered it?

ICSI – intracytoplasmic sperm injection – is a way of enabling couples to conceive where the man has little and/or poor quality sperm, by injecting a single sperm into an egg. Any resulting embryos are then transferred into the uterus by IVF. You may be offered it:

- if your partner produces no sperm (azoospermia), for example, because of blockage or absence of the vas deferens, the tube that transports sperm from the testes.
- if sperm quality is so poor that conception is unlikely.
- if you have tried IVF but none or few of the eggs have fertilised.
- if a sperm analysis shows the presence of anti-sperm antibodies.

What will the procedure involve?

Your ovaries will be stimulated and eggs collected in exactly the same way as for IVF. Your partner will be asked to produce a semen sample on the same day your eggs are collected. This will be prepared and the best sperm picked out using a needle. A second sample may be needed if the first did not yield enough suitable sperm. Alternatively, sperm will be aspirated (see p.85) using a fine needle under local anaesthetic, or surgically retrieved under general anaesthetic by one of several techniques described on p.85 and frozen until it is needed.

What happens next?

A single sperm is selected under the microscope and immobilised so it cannot swim out of the egg once it has been injected. This is then carefully loaded into an extremely thin glass needle. The eggs are then stripped of their surrounding cells using an artificial enzyme (similar to that which sperm normally produce to allow penetration) and held in position while the embryologist injects a single sperm into the egg. Once fertilised, the eggs are allowed to develop (as for IVF) and the most viable embryos chosen before being transferred to the womb.

How many eggs will fertilise and will any of them be damaged?

Because a needle is injected into the egg, there is a risk of damaging it. It's estimated that around 10–15 per cent will be damaged even in the hands of an experienced embryologist, although some eggs are more fragile and damage more easily. Around 50–60 per cent of mature eggs usually fertilise following ICSI.

Are there any risks?

ICSI is still a relatively new treatment and its long-term safety is still not fully established. Studies suggest that there is a slightly increased risk of chromosomal abnormalities (around 0.9 per cent compared with a usual level of 0.6 per cent in children born after normal conception or traditional IVF). It has been found that in cases of severe male infertility, some men have a defect in their Y chromosome, known as a microdeletion, in which a small part of the chromosome is missing or absent. This defect will be passed on to any male babies. If you conceive using ICSI, you'll need to think carefully about whether to have prenatal screening tests such as amniocentesis to check for any potential abnormalities.

What is SUZI?

Sub-zonal insemination was a forerunner of ICSI. Rather than injecting a single sperm into the egg, the sperm is injected into the perivitelline space between the egg and shell.

ISSUES TO CONSIDER

The fertility clinic just doesn't tell me what's going on with my treatment. What can I do?

Every clinic should provide written information and keep you informed throughout your treatment about exactly what is being done and why. After each cycle you should have the opportunity to review your treatment with the doctor and decide how to proceed. Make a note of any questions you want to ask before each visit and ensure that your questions are answered in a way that you understand. Bear in mind that English may not be your consultant's first language, or that information may have to be repeated or written down until you are completely sure of what you are being told.

What if I'm not happy with my treatment?

If you are being treated in an NHS hospital, there are established complaints procedures:

- In the first instance you may want to raise the complaint informally with the person concerned. Your counsellor may be able to suggest a way to do this. Many complaints can be resolved quickly in this way.

- If you don't feel able to complain directly or if you want to make a formal complaint, you can phone NHS Direct on 0845 4647 or go to www.nhs.direct.nhs.uk. They will tell you how to complain and can put you in touch with someone who can help you.

- You could also approach your local Patient Advisory and Liaison Service (PALS), who will help you draft a letter and, if you agree, can arrange a meeting to try to resolve matters and/or put you in touch with the hospital's Complaints Manager, who can carry out further investigations on your behalf.

- If you are still unhappy, the Complaints Manager, or PALS, can put you in touch with a convener. This is an independent, specially trained person who can review your complaint and may decide to set up an independent review panel. The panel will talk to all concerned and produce a short report setting out its findings and other comments or suggestions, which will be sent both to you and the hospital's Chief Executive.

- If you still aren't happy, you can take your case to the Ombudsman (Health Service Commissioner), an independent person appointed by Parliament. For details write to the Health Service Commissioner for England, 11th Floor, Millbank Tower, London SW1P 4QP Tel: 0845 015 4033, www.health.ombudsman.org.uk.

How do I make a complaint about a private clinic?

Although the clinic may employ an official Complaints Manager, there is no clear-cut complaints procedure within the private sector. Consultants working in the private sector are not usually employed directly by the clinic, so you will need to find out what the procedure is for making a complaint. If your complaint is about a different aspect of your care, such as the quality or cost of treatment, you may need to complain to several different people. Private hospitals and clinics are regulated by the Registered Homes Act 1984 and must be registered with the health authority. If you aren't happy with the response to your complaint, you can complain to the health authority, although they won't deal with clinical complaints (ie about a doctor or treatment). If your complaint is serious, you may decide to withhold payment. Be aware that the doctor or clinic could sue you for recovery, so it would be a good idea to seek legal advice first. If your complaint isn't resolved to your satisfaction there isn't an independent watchdog so you may have to resort to legal action.

I don't feel able to complain about my treatment while in the middle of an IVF cycle, can I get help with this?

You may want to talk to your counsellor, who may be able to help you decide if and when you should go ahead with your complaint. Alternatively you may want to phone the ISSUE helpline, which is staffed by counsellors who are experienced in helping people with a wide range of issues to do with fertility treatment. It is important to complain if you feel you have been treated unfairly at whatever point in your treatment. Those providing your healthcare need to know your views and complaining should never affect your treatment or the services you can expect.

Some questions to consider:
- Who or what are you complaining about?
- If you are complaining about a person, where do they work?
- Who do they work for?
- When did the thing you are complaining about happen?
- What are your main concerns?
- What do you hope to achieve – An apology? An explanation? Action to put things right? Compensation?

How do I find out about alternative treatments/clinics?

If you are unhappy with your treatment and think you would like to be treated in a different clinic, you can use the information at the back of this guide to compare units. In addition, you can use the HFEA guide and the various materials produced by infertility support organisations such as CHILD and ISSUE and websites such as FertilityConfidential. ISSUE's newsletter includes first-hand accounts of members' personal experiences of different clinics.

Waiting for results

Waiting for the results of treatment is possibly the most stressful time of all. Most clinics will encourage you to perform a pregnancy test yourself two weeks after gametes or embryos are transferred. The test detects the levels of the early pregnancy hormone hCG and most pregnancy testing kits are pretty accurate. However, hCG increases dramatically in the first few weeks of pregnancy, so if you get a negative result or only a weakly positive one, you may want to carry out another test a few days later. After this, you should have your pregnancy confirmed by a test at the clinic.

What does a 'low positive' pregnancy test result mean?
Pregnancy can be detected by doing a blood test for hCG, although this is not performed as routinely in fertility clinics in the UK as in America. If a low level is found, it may be described as a low positive result. hCG levels vary tremendously between different women, so a low positive result doesn't necessarily mean that your pregnancy is insecure. However, hCG can also be present after an early pregnancy loss, or a pregnancy that failed to begin or implant properly. For this reason, many experts recommend delaying doing an hCG blood test until three days after missing a period. If you have had an hCG injection as part of your treatment, the hormone will take from five to 14 days to clear from your system. This can cause problems with interpreting pregnancy tests done within this time, so it may be better to wait another couple of weeks before having a blood test done.

How am I likely to feel after a successful treatment?
It is common to feel many conflicting emotions: happy one minute, doubtful and afraid the next. If a treatment cycle results in a pregnancy, you may well feel elated and amazed that you have finally conceived after all the tests and treatment. On the other hand, you may experience a sense of anti-climax and possible anxiety over what your pregnancy might hold and whether you will carry your baby to term. Try to accept your feelings, whatever they are. Most pregnant women, however they have conceived,

experience a mixture of different feelings as they begin to take on the reality of having a child. If you have conceived as a result of fertility treatment, you may feel that you are now just an ordinary pregnant woman rather than an infertility 'patient'. It can be difficult, especially if you have been trying to conceive for some time without success, to make the psychological leap from one to the other. Having had such extensive and intensive contact with the medical system, you may even feel rather bereft of the attention you have previously received from the doctors and nurses now that your – and their – desired end has been achieved. Talking to your counsellor or seeking help from one of the fertility charities such as ACeBabes (see p.265) can help you deal with the common anxieties that happen in pregnancy following assisted conception.

What steps do I need to take if I am pregnant?

Once your pregnancy has been confirmed, you will need to make arrangements for your antenatal care. The first step is to visit your GP, who will take down some initial details. They will arrange a 'booking' visit at the hospital. Here you will meet the obstetrician who will be responsible for your care during pregnancy and birth, and the midwives who will be involved in your routine antenatal care. This visit is an opportunity for you to discuss where you want to give birth, what type of birth you are hoping for and what antenatal tests may be recommended. Antenatal care usually doesn't start until around the twelfth week of pregnancy. During this time you may feel particularly insecure and in need of support. Some fertility clinics will encourage you to stay in contact during this time and may suggest you talk to your counsellor and/or any support group. The clinic may also be able to put you in touch with other women who have had a baby after fertility treatment who will know how you are feeling in these early weeks.

What support will the clinic give me? Will they give me a six-week scan?

This will vary a lot. Some clinics will remain in touch with you in the early weeks of pregnancy (before you get into the antenatal care system) and will do a six-week ultrasound scan to check the baby's health and development (although you may have to pay for this).

Some will also do an eight-week scan to check for any abnormalities. Ask the clinic what sort of support there will be if you do become pregnant and if you are paying for your treatment, is this included.

Will the clinic have links with a maternity unit?
If your fertility treatment was carried out in large NHS hospital (even if you paid for private treatment) or in a large private hospital, there may well be links with the hospital's maternity unit and your notes will be available. If you had your treatment in a private clinic dealing solely with infertility, it may have links with maternity units or the clinic itself may provide a certain amount of support and care. If the clinic has no links with a maternity service, it will be up to you to tell the doctors and midwives caring for you that you conceived as a result of fertility treatment.

Will my pregnancy be the same as if I'd conceived 'naturally'?
All things being equal, your pregnancy should be the same as if you had conceived naturally, although there may be other factors that put you into a high-risk group. In this case, your care will be tailored to your individual needs. You may well need to have more of your antenatal care at the hospital, or more appointments with the consultant. Your risk will depend on:
- Your previous reproductive history (infertility treatment, number of previous pregnancies, any miscarriages and/or stillbirths).
- Your age.
- Whether you are expecting more than one baby.
- Your overall health.

Emotionally, you may find it tougher than a woman who has conceived naturally and it may be wise to alert the midwives and doctors caring for you that you have had fertility treatment.

Will my baby be normal?
All medical procedures carry risks as well as benefits, as do 'natural' pregnancy and birth. There is a one to two per cent risk that any baby – however conceived – may have an abnormality. Many millions of normal babies have been born worldwide as a result of fertility treatment, and many studies have been done – most of which have found no evidence of any adverse effect on their health. Two recent

studies published in the New England Journal of Medicine claim that there is an increased risk of birth defects and low birth weight in babies conceived as a result of assisted conception. Some studies also show that babies born as a result of ICSI may have a slightly increased risk of chromosomal abnormalities, although research is as yet conflicting and inconclusive. It is important to bear in mind that these studies are being questioned, the absolute risk of having a baby with a birth defect is still relatively low and that assisted conception offers you a 90–95 per cent chance of having a healthy baby.

What is prenatal testing and am I likely to need it?
Prenatal testing involves a number of different procedures used to check the health of the developing fetus. Tests include:

- **Blood tests** A number of these can be performed which measure the presence of various chemicals and give an indication of the risk of abnormalities including Down's syndrome or spina bifida.
- **Amniocentesis** in which a small amount of amniotic fluid is withdrawn and tested for abnormalities such as Down's syndrome and other chromosomal disorders.
- **Chorionic villus sampling (CVS)** in which a small sample of the chorionic tissue is taken from the edge of the placenta and analysed for chromosomal abnormalities.
- **Nuchal fold scan** in which an ultrasound scan is performed on the back of the baby's neck (the nuchal fold). This can, with other indicators, suggest that the baby has a risk of Down's syndrome.

All women will have to decide whether to have prenatal testing and which tests to have. It can be a difficult decision for any woman but particularly so if you have conceived as a result of fertility treatment, because both amniocentesis and CVS carry a small risk of causing miscarriage. On the other hand, you have to consider how you would feel if your baby was born with a chromosomal abnormality.

MULTIPLE PREGNANCY

What if it's a multiple pregnancy?
The consultant who is in charge of your antenatal care will want to monitor you carefully throughout pregnancy to ensure that you and your babies remain healthy and that the babies are delivered at the best

time for your and their well-being. You can get more information about the management of multiple pregnancy from TAMBA (see p.266).

Why does fertility treatment result in so many multiple births?
The more embryos or eggs transferred, the greater the risk of becoming pregnant with twins or triplets. Even when just one embryo is transferred it may split in two, resulting in identical twins, or if two are transferred, either or both may split, resulting in triplets or even quadruplets. Even the use of ovulation induction, without assisted conception, can increase the likelihood of multiple pregnancy.

What are my chances of becoming pregnant with twins or triplets?
Research suggests that when only one embryo is transferred, the number of multiple pregnancies is less than five per cent, of which one per cent are triplet pregnancies – around the same as in a 'natural' conception. When two embryos are transferred, the number of twin pregnancies increases to almost 25 per cent, although there is little change in the number of women who conceive triplets. When three embryos are transferred (the maximum number permitted by the HFEA), the risk of triplets increases to six per cent, depending on factors including your age, the quality of the embryos and the number of previous attempts.

What are the dangers associated with multiple pregnancy?
- The rate of miscarriage is higher, as is the risk of pre-eclampsia (high blood pressure during pregnancy).
- Babies are more likely to be born early and by Caesarean section.
- Babies are more likely to be below normal birthweight and the risk of physical and mental problems ie cerebral palsy is increased.

If I am pregnant with twins or triplets, will I be offered a selective termination?
The increased incidence of multiple pregnancy caused by assisted conception has resulted in an increase in selective termination. This involves injecting the heart of the selected fetus with a toxic fluid, a procedure that can only be done after eight weeks of pregnancy.

Some doctors will not carry out selective termination following fertility treatment, as long as you and the fetuses are healthy. If you are pregnant with triplets or more (for example, if you have had treatment abroad that allows the transfer of more than three embryos), the doctor will take your and your fetuses' health into account. They will also consider how having three or more babies is likely to affect you and the rest of your family.

Selective termination is one of the many complex and difficult issues thrown up by new reproductive technology. It is an undeniably difficult choice to be faced with, especially when you have gone through so much to get pregnant, and you will need advice and support to help you decide. As well as discussing it with your consultant and your partner, you may wish to talk to the counsellor at the clinic to try to come to a decision that you think will be right for you.

What factors should I take into account if the doctor suggests selective termination?

- Your general health and how a multiple pregnancy and birth is likely to affect this.
- How you feel you will cope physically and emotionally with a multiple pregnancy.
- How you will cope physically and emotionally once the babies are born (eg how much help and support are you likely to have? how many other children do you have, and how does a multiple pregnancy affect them and your financial situation?).
- How you might cope with the emotional consequences of a termination and with the small but nevertheless real risk of losing the other fetuses as well.
- Whether you have any strong religious beliefs or ethical concerns that affect your feelings about termination.

MISCARRIAGE

Am I more likely to miscarry after assisted conception?
There is a risk of miscarriage in any pregnancy, however you have conceived. Eight to 10 per cent of pregnancies achieved following a 'natural' conception end in a miscarriage. After IVF treatment, the

Christine Butcher, 39

I started trying to conceive when I was almost 38. I'd had a few problems with irregular bleeding so I was concerned about how easy it would be. After trying for less than a year I went to my GP, who referred me for a laparoscopy. There was a six-month wait on the NHS so I had the operation privately. It turned out that I had fibroids but the NHS gynaecologist didn't think that was the problem and diagnosed unexplained infertility. However, the private gynaecologist thought I should try IVF.

Initially, I referred myself to the IVF unit at the local hospital and I was seen within three weeks. The clinic was very pessimistic, telling me that IVF was not very successful and that the fibroids would halve my chances of success. I was seeing an acupuncturist at the time and she suggested the IVF hospital we eventually chose. They have a 41 per cent live birth rate, which is the highest in the country. Unusually, they put three embryos back for women over 35, which is controversial. I was very nervous about this but they told us it was our best chance of success. I conceived after the first cycle, but I had a low positive pregnancy test and when I went back a week later it was negative.

I waited another six months, during which I did the Foresight pre-conceptual programme. The gynaecologist said they suspected a blood flow problem and to my amazement put me on Viagra (it apparently helps to get more blood to the uterus). As soon as they replaced the embryos they put me on heparin and aspirin, which stops blood clotting (another reason why some women are thought to miscarry) and this time I conceived twins. Unfortunately, I miscarried one of them and I then had to decide whether to discontinue the aspirin and heparin.

I was worried I might lose the other baby if I continued so I asked the Multiple Birth Foundation to recommend a private specialist for a second opinion. The private specialist did a clotting test and said that I didn't have a clotting problem so I came off it. The obstetrician I was seeing on the NHS was supportive of my decision to get a second opinion, even though it meant bypassing the NHS.

I am now 30 weeks pregnant, although I had a threatened miscarriage at 22 weeks. I am constantly monitored at the NHS clinic and I am scanned regularly by a high-risk pregnancy specialist. I also go to the day assessment unit for regular checks.

Emotionally, the IVF has been relatively easy, but the pregnancy has been harrowing. The fertility clinic has been very supportive and positive and I think that makes a huge difference. I felt that the local hospital was unnecessarily negative. I haven't taken up the offer of counselling as I didn't feel I needed it. I've been very open with my friends, family and work colleagues and I have made contact with women from all over the world through the Internet. When I lost the twin, the women on the website gave me hope. Initially my obstetrician was fairly negative and thought it would be a disaster. The next time I went to see him, he said he'd done some research and that he was more positive.

My advice to other people embarking on fertility treatment is not to expect quick results. You need to shop around for the best clinic and not to be afraid to ask lots of searching questions. At the same time it's important to be realistic. The whole thing is very tough, but I feel in the end it will have been well worth it.

risk is around 15 per cent. The slight increase is thought to be due to the fact that the risk of miscarriage rises with age, and that women who have assisted conception are usually older, on average, than those who conceive naturally.

How will I know if I'm miscarrying?

The first sign is likely to be bleeding from the vagina. This may be pinkish or brown in colour, often around the time when a period would have been due. If the bleeding is slight and painless, it may be a threatened miscarriage (see below). In a true miscarriage, bleeding continues and becomes heavier, bright red in colour and is accompanied by clots and cramping pains as the uterus contracts to expel the fetus. A tiny embryo or fetus may be visible and/or what doctors call the 'products' of conception – blood clots and tissue from the placenta, membranes and the lining of the uterus. The longer bleeding and cramping continues, the more likely it is you are having a miscarriage. If the doctor performs an internal examination, the cervix will be open (dilated). You will usually be admitted to hospital for observation, an ultrasound scan and blood and urine tests to see whether you are still pregnant and whether the pregnancy is viable. If it is not (ie if the fetus has died) the bleeding will stop when the uterus has completely expelled the fetus, or following a D&C (see p.119) to clear out the uterus.

What is a threatened miscarriage? Is there anything I can do about it?

A threatened miscarriage is the term used when there is a bloodstained discharge from the vagina during the first few weeks of pregnancy. This may last anything from a few days to a few weeks and there may be some pain or cramping. The doctor will probably advise you to rest in bed until the bleeding stops, although activity does not cause miscarriage. In a threatened miscarriage, if the doctor performs an internal examination, the cervix will be tightly shut. An ultrasound scan may also be done to check whether the baby is alive. One in five women experiences bleeding in early pregnancy so threatened miscarriage is relatively common.

What is a missed miscarriage?

This is when a miscarriage happens (the fetus or embryo dies in the womb) but there are no symptoms (such as bleeding) and the fetus is not lost naturally. It may be suspected if your symptoms such as breast tenderness and nausea disappear or you simply may not 'feel pregnant' any more. It may also be detected on a routine antenatal examination if the uterus has not grown in size. If there is any doubt, an ultrasound scan will be performed to check for the presence or absence of the baby's heartbeat. Sometimes this may need to be repeated and a pregnancy urine test done.

When is miscarriage most likely to take place?

Most miscarriages happen before the twelfth week of pregnancy (bearing in mind that pregnancy is dated from the first day of your last menstrual period and not from conception). It is thought that as many as half of all miscarriages occur even before the embryo implants in the uterus – that is, before most women who have conceived 'naturally' are even aware they are pregnant. In the early days after the embryo implants in the uterus – but still before pregnancy is clinically recognised – the miscarriage rate is around 30 per cent. Once pregnancy is clinically recognised – that is between days 35 and 50 following conception – another quarter of fetuses are miscarried. The risk of miscarriage declines after 12 weeks and becomes progressively less likely as pregnancy continues.

Is there any way to prevent a miscarriage?

Miscarriage is normally due to chance and there is not usually any way to prevent it. However, you may feel better if you take a few steps to ensure that you are in good overall health before attempting to become pregnant again by making sure that your diet is healthy, that you reduce your alcohol limit and take regular exercise, avoid stress where possible and that your weight is normal for your height and build. You are more likely to miscarry following IVF if you are overweight. You should also be sure to take 0.4mg folic acid daily to reduce the risk of spina bifida and other neural tube defects. You may want to take particular care at the time your period would have been due and to avoid sex and strenuous exercise during the first few weeks (although there is no evidence that these cause miscarriage).

Why do miscarriages happen?

It's natural to want to find a reason why you miscarried but in many cases it is simply bad luck. Miscarriage is more common if you are over 35 and have taken six months or more to conceive and if you have had a previous miscarriage. Known causes include existing diseases such as diabetes, heart problems, kidney disorders, systemic lupus (an autoimmune disease) and abnormalities of the pelvic organs. Other possible reasons include:

- Chromosomal problems: the most common cause of miscarriage is a chromosomal abnormality that causes disturbed cell division following fertilisation. The embryo is unable to develop further and is expelled by the uterus.
- Genetic disease: in rarer instances you or your partner may be a carrier of a faulty gene, such as cystic fibrosis, which results in recurrent miscarriage.
- Hormonal problems: eg increased production of LH as in PCOS.
- Auto-immune abnormalities: eg antiphospholipid syndrome.
- Infection: eg chlamydia or other sexually transmitted infections.
- Incompetent cervix: when the cervix starts to open early. This is more usually a cause of later miscarriage (ie after 12 weeks).
- Abnormalities of the structure of the uterus or problems such as polyps or fibroids, which mean that the fetus can't grow properly.

Will the cause of my miscarriage be investigated?

If you miscarry after assisted conception, an investigation as to why it happened is unlikely, unless there are particular reasons to be suspicious. A large number of women miscarry and many do so more than once. After three or more miscarriages, the doctor may suggest some investigations to try and find out why (see below).

How am I likely to feel if I miscarry?

Any kind of loss can lead to feelings of grief, guilt, anger and depression. It can be particularly hard to miscarry when you want a baby so much and have jumped through so many hoops to try and have one. If you have not told people you were receiving fertility treatment, or not told those around you were pregnant, it can be especially difficult trying to behave normally and keep your feelings to yourself. Talking to your counsellor or contacting a support group such as the Miscarriage Association (see p.265) (who may be able to put you in touch with another woman who has experienced a miscarriage or miscarriages) may help you come to terms with your loss.

Will I need to have a D&C?

A D&C (dilatation and curettage – or evacuation) may be performed to clear out your uterus and help prevent prolonged bleeding and/or infection. This will possibly be carried out under a general anaesthetic and may mean an overnight stay in hospital. However, a D&C will not weaken your cervix or increase your likelihood of miscarrying in a future pregnancy.

What if I keep having miscarriages?

Recurrent miscarriage is a factor in subfertility. If you have three or more miscarriages, your fertility specialist may perform tests to see why you keep miscarrying and/or may refer you to a special recurrent miscarriage clinic. Tests may include:

- Blood tests for hormone levels eg FSH (high levels can indicate that you are in the run-up to the menopause) and LH.
- Blood tests for auto-antibodies. Antibodies are produced by the body's immune system and may destroy eggs, sperm or embryos, rather like someone who has a transplant and rejects it. In particular, antibodies called antiphospholipids and anticardiolipids are linked to blood clotting in early pregnancy and slow growth of the fetus. Two blood tests done at least eight weeks apart can detect if levels of these are persistently raised. If so, you will be diagnosed with primary phospholipid antibody syndrome and treated with low-dose aspirin and heparin injections to minimise the risk of miscarriage. Untreated, the risk of miscarriage is 90 per cent; treatment reduces the risk to 25–30 per cent.
- Ultrasound scan to check that the uterus is a normal shape.
- Checking the chromosomes of the embryo to see if there are any genetic abnormalities passed on by you or your partner. This is not funded by the NHS so you will have to pay for it.
- If your consultant can find no apparent reason as to why you keep miscarrying, they may refer you to a doctor with a special interest in recurrent miscarriage for further investigation.

What is an ectopic pregnancy and does fertility treatment put me at greater risk of having one?

This is also known as extrauterine or tubal pregnancy. The embryo begins to grow outside the uterus, often in the fallopian tube but sometimes in the ovary, cervix or elsewhere in the abdomen. If your fertility problems are a result of tubal blockage or damage (see p.59), your risk of an ectopic pregnancy is around four to five per cent.

How does ectopic pregnancy happen?

If embryos were transferred into the fallopian tube using GIFT, they may not travel into the uterus (for this reason you should not be offered GIFT if your tubes are unhealthy or damaged). Even if embryos were inserted into the womb, they can sometimes migrate upwards and become implanted in a fallopian tube. An early scan and pregnancy hormone level checks can detect ectopic pregnancy at an early stage so it can be treated immediately.

How will I know if I have an ectopic pregnancy?

Symptoms include low abdominal pain and vaginal bleeding which may be dark brown in colour. You may be given a vaginal ultrasound scan to check whether there is a fetus in your uterus, swelling in the fallopian tube or blood in the abdominal cavity. Taking repeated blood tests for the presence of hCG (see p.108) can help confirm diagnosis. If the doctor does think you have an ectopic pregnancy, you will be given a laparoscopy to check, after which your fallopian tube may need to be removed. It may be possible to conserve the tube by removing the fetus and reconstituting the tube surgically, or by injecting the tube with a special drug that will destroy the fetus.

WHEN TREATMENT FAILS

After unsuccessful treatment, you and your partner will naturally be extremely disappointed and may want to take some time to give yourself a chance to recuperate before you decide whether you want to try again and, if so, how and when. You will have a follow-up appointment with your consultant to talk over what happened and to work through the treatment cycle: your response to the drugs, eggs and/or sperm collection, fertilisation and whether any more tests need to be done,although this will usually not be necessary unless something abnormal was picked up (like a polyp) during the cycle. You should discuss whether a further attempt is worth trying and if anything can be done to improve your chances, should you decide to try again. You may also want to seek counselling (see p.150).

Will the consultant be able to offer an explanation?

Sometimes the reasons for unsuccessful treatment may be clear and the consultant will be able to discuss this with you. However, just as with a naturally occurring conception, many pregnancies are lost at an early stage. These early 'miscarriages' usually pass unnoticed or are dismissed as a 'late period' in women who are not having fertility treatment. However, if you have had treatment, you may be acutely aware that you have conceived and then miscarried. It's important to remember that the chances of conceiving in any one menstrual cycle are no more than 20–30 per cent, even in a fertile couple.

Why might assisted conception fail?

The most common reason for it to fail, as with a 'natural' pregnancy, is because of poor embryo quality. The egg may not have matured properly in the first place, it may not have divided properly following fertilisation and many apparently healthy-looking embryos have chromosomal abnormalities. The quality control tests described in the previous chapter allow doctors to choose healthier, potentially more viable embryos and so these problems may become less common in future. Despite this, some pregnancies fail even when the quality of the embryos was considered to be very high. Research has found that women who have poor blood flow to the uterus have a lower chance of conceiving and a higher risk of miscarrying if they do conceive. The state of the fallopian tubes and uterus is important too.

Is there anything I can do to improve my chances next time?

Chances are that you are doing all that you can to stay healthy: eating a nutritious diet, taking sufficient exercise, taking folic acid, and avoiding alcohol and/or smoking. Many fertility specialists believe that the best thing you can do is to try and relax. You may want to take a short break if you can afford it, or do something more proactive such as seeking complementary treatment (see p.66), as many of these act by helping you to relax. Whilst there is very little statistical evidence that they can help improve fertility, there is much anecdotal evidence that it can help, not least by restoring a much-needed sense of control that is often lost when you are undergoing intensive medical treatment.

How long should I wait before trying again?

Most fertility experts recommend waiting a couple of menstrual cycles to allow your body time to recover, to give you some time off from the stress of infertility treatment and to allow you to come to terms with having had an unsuccessful treatment.

What is the maximum number of IVF treatments I can have?

Every consultant will have a different opinion as to how many treatments you should have. If you have managed to get treatment funded by the NHS, this will usually be limited. If you are paying for private treatment, there is theoretically no limit on the number of attempts – other than your emotional and physical ability to cope with repeated disappointment and the size of your purse. Bear in mind that although the chances of success increase with each cycle, they level off at around the eighth cycle and thereafter start to fall.

When should I give up on assisted conception?

Whether you have had just one or numerous attempts, it's important to remember that you always have choices. One is to stop treatment and/or consider other ways of having a child. This may be the point when you can no longer afford it – but even if you aren't paying for treatment, you may feel that you can no longer stand the emotional strain. Your consultant may advise that you have little or no chance of conceiving. If you do decide to stop, it's important to feel that it is your choice. Stopping does not mean that you are a failure, that you haven't done enough or that you have to give up all hope of having a child. It may mean exploring surrogacy, adoption or fostering. For some it will mean deciding that, having given it your best shot, you now want to move on and make a child free life. Every couple will come to their own decision in their own way and their own time. There are no right or wrong choices – just the one that is best for you.

Donor assisted conception

Donor conception is the process by which you are helped to conceive using sperm, eggs (or in some cases, embryos) donated by another man and/or woman. This may be used with or without IVF and other assisted conception techniques. In the next section, we tell you which clinics offer egg donation. You can also use the HFEA list. The National Gamete Donation Trust website (www.ngdt.org.uk) also lists relevant clinics and their contact details.

Some doctors present donor assisted conception, especially sperm donation, as something to be tried when everything else has failed. Some couples also feel that the procedure is something they are only prepared to contemplate when all other avenues have been exhausted. However, in many circumstances, the situation is not clear-cut. Some women over 40 who have had several attempts at IVF and who have a statistical chance – albeit slim – of conceiving using their own eggs, may decide to use donor eggs. This gives them a higher chance of getting pregnant but a lower risk of having a baby with an abnormality (as the eggs used are from women under 35). In fact, some women say that once the pressure to 'beat the clock' is removed in this way, they feel much less stressed about the whole business. Others who have the risk of passing on a genetic or chromosomal illness or condition may decide that egg or sperm donation is the best option.

Donor assisted conception is quite different to other forms of assisted conception in the sense that it raises unique implications for you, your partner and both of your families. For this reason, it is worth taking plenty of time to explore the different issues thoroughly before making up your mind to go ahead.

In what circumstances might we consider donor conception?
If you are a woman and:
- you were born with poor ovarian function or have gone through an early menopause (premature ovarian failure).
- you have no ovaries or have had your ovaries removed (oophorectomy) eg as part of cancer treatment.

- there is a high risk of passing on, or giving birth to a baby with a chromosomal or genetic abnormality.
- you are ovulating normally but the quality and quantity of your eggs is poor because of your age.
- repeated attempts at IVF have failed as a result of poor quality/quantity of eggs.
- you have no response or a poor response to fertility drugs.
- you have had recurrent unexplained miscarriages.
- you have ROS, your periods have always been irregular or absent and tests have revealed low oestrogen and high FSH levels.
- you are single or without a male partner and want to have a baby (sperm donation).

If you are a man and:
- you aren't producing any sperm (azoospermia).
- you have had a vasectomy or a failed vasectomy reversal.
- you have poor sperm quality.
- your sperm has failed to fertilise an egg in IVF and/or ICSI.
- you have a high risk of passing on a chromosomal or genetic disease or condition that is passed down the male line.

What are the chances of success?

A number of different factors can affect success but live birth rates compare well with those achieved by IVF and, in the case of egg donation, are often higher. This is because the eggs are donated by women under 35 and so are usually of better quality. The following statistics will give you an idea of success rates:

- With Donor insemination (DI), the overall live birth rate is around 10 per cent per cycle, although this can vary from 1.8 per cent to 19.2 per cent according to the most recent HFEA guide. If the female partner is under 38, the rate is higher – around 10.6 per cent compared to around three or four per cent in women aged 40 and over.
- With egg donation, the likelihood of getting pregnant is around 20–25 per cent per treatment cycle, slightly higher than with conventional IVF.
- With embryo donation, the live birth rate is around 20–25 per cent per treatment cycle.

What issues do we need to consider before taking this route?

Infertility is a minefield of complicated emotional and moral decisions with long-term implications for you, your child and the rest of your family. However, donor assisted conception poses more than most. The decision to use a donor is far from easy and each couple and/or individual must come to the decision that is right for them in their own time. Deciding to take the donor route is not just the next logical step in treatment. There are no right or wrong answers, but the following are some issues you might want to consider.

Using donor eggs

- Why do you feel using a donated egg or sperm is a better choice for you than surrogacy, adoption or life without a child?
- If using an anonymous donor, how do you feel about the child having half the genetic characteristics of someone else's family?
- How do you feel about the fact that either you or your partner will not be your child's genetic parent?
- How would you feel about not knowing the donor? How would you feel about knowing the donor?
- How would you feel knowing that other children may be born from the same donor and that your child may have half-siblings?
- How does the idea of donor assisted conception fit with your religious and/or ethical views?
- Have you talked to your family about the idea that you might use donated eggs or sperm? If not, why? If so, what was their reaction?
- Who will you/should you tell and when (your parents, close family members, close friends, your GP)? Research suggests that children are more well balanced if their origins are not kept secret but shared with at least close family, friends and the child.
- What will you tell other friends and relatives, if anything?
- What will you tell your child about his or her origins?

Who can I talk things through with?

Firstly, you and your partner will want to make sure that you both feel comfortable with the decision to choose donor assisted conception. At your initial visit to the clinic, the consultant should explain what the procedure involves and discuss social, ethical and legal issues with you. You should also be given an opportunity to talk to the counsellor at the clinic to explore the complex psychological issues and feelings that are involved and to discuss the implications of practicalities like HIV testing. The HFEA specifies that all couples having donation should be counselled at least once. The clinic can put you in touch with its own counsellor, or you can find one through BICA. Some couples have fears that anxieties expressed to a counsellor at the fertility clinic may prejudice their chances of treatment. Seeing a completely independent counsellor can give you more privacy and increased freedom of expression. Some clinics go out of their way to make sure the counsellors they use operate independently (see p.x151). If you have strong religious beliefs, you may want to discuss the issues involved with a priest or other leader.

Are there any helpful support groups?

The National Gamete Donation Trust (see p.266) raises awareness of the national shortage of sperm, egg and embryo donors. The Donor Conception Network (see p.265) was set up solely to help would-be and actual gamete donation parents think about the issues surrounding the use of egg or sperm donation to found families. They offer support from diagnosis onwards and through the long haul of parenting. ACeBabes (see p.265) provides support for anyone using assisted conception and has a subgroup for those who have used donor conception. Daisy Network (see p.265) is a support group for women who have gone through premature menopause and provides information about egg donation. It can be very helpful to talk to someone who has had experience of donor-assisted conception and of bringing up children conceived in this way, and the last three of these groups will be able to put you in touch with someone.

Should we tell our family and friends?

Even if you have not found it difficult to talk about your fertility problems, it can be hard to talk about donor assisted conception. However, if you do not tell anyone, you may feel extremely isolated. Many parents who have children born as a result of egg, sperm or embryo donation believe it is high time that the veil of secrecy surrounding donor conception was removed, as shame, fear and deception are not a good basis on which to build family life. Most of those who have taken the plunge have been pleasantly surprised by the positive reactions they have received.

Should we delay joining a waiting list until we are completely sure we want to go ahead?

In an ideal world you would be completely sure before going ahead with a decision to use donor assisted conception. The reality is that you may not feel totally certain that you have made the right decision until after your child is born. Given the length of waiting lists, many people with experience of donor assisted conception advise going on a list while you sort your feelings out to avoid undue delays. However, the Donor Conception Network points out that because the wait is likely to be shorter for donated sperm, couples are advised not to start this treatment until both partners have had the opportunity to really understand what they are doing. Couples waiting for an egg donor have a longer (often very frustrating) period to integrate the issues involved into their lives. Because the baby is nurtured inside the recipient mother, she has nine months to accept and adapt to the fact that her child is not genetically connected to her. In this case, it is probably better to get onto a waiting list as soon as possible.

If I conceive using a donated egg, will I feel as if I'm carrying another woman's baby?

This is a common fear. The majority of women who have conceived using donor eggs say that once they are actually pregnant, any feeling that the baby is 'not really theirs' disappears. Counselling can help you work through any difficult feelings you may have.

If I conceive using donor sperm, will it matter that it won't be my partner's baby genetically?

If you are in a long-term loving relationship, having a baby is about giving birth to a child that you and your partner have created. When you discover that this will never happen, after the first feelings of overwhelming shock, you may experience disappointment, sadness or anger. You may worry that your feelings for your partner will change, that you won't find him attractive any more and you may find it difficult to have sex knowing there is no chance of conceiving.

You need to give yourself – and your partner – time to come to terms with the implications of this in your own way. Many women who have conceived using donor sperm say that the process of insemination with a stranger's sperm can feel strange. Some even feel

Jane Moorcock

In August 1998, after some months of investigation and no clear explanation of why I wasn't getting pregnant, the consultant at the private clinic I'd chosen decided to put me on a three-month course of Clomid. Unfortunately, nothing happened so we found ourselves back there again three months later. This time, we were advised to try IUI (intra-uterine insemination) as that's the least complicated treatment cycle for what was then being described as a case of 'unexplained' infertility. By that stage, we'd been trying to conceive for about two years and the only factor indicating that there might really be something wrong was that my FSH levels were higher than they should have been.

IUI was less stressful than I'd anticipated. I thought I wouldn't be able to cope with injecting myself with drugs but then I was given an injector 'pen', which meant all I had to do was press a button and I didn't even have to watch the needle going into my thigh. I was lucky that the drugs didn't make me feel ill and that there was a bus that took me all the way to the hospital door for my early morning scans and blood tests. I produced three good-sized follicles and on the day of the actual insemination the nurses were very positive, chatting away about how I'd cope with a brand-new baby and the postgraduate course I'd just signed up for.

Unfortunately, all the optimism was misplaced. After two weeks of desperately trying to distract myself and think about anything other than children, my period started. To me, there seemed to be some irony in the fact that the day we were due to do the pregnancy test was 14 February.

So now it was a question of what to do next. Every blood test revealed an even higher FSH level, making us panic that time was running out. It seemed as though we had no choice but to try IVF. The only trouble was, my body didn't seem ready to cope with IVF. Twice I injected myself with drugs and then went along to scans where I was told that I'd responded well to the suppressant drugs but not at all to the stimulants. Twice the cycle was cancelled. The only option left to us seemed to be egg donation. The trouble with egg donation was that not only did it involve a whole new set of issues, it also meant further delay while we looked for a donor. The clinic we were using then had a five-year waiting list and recommended we should go elsewhere. We put our names down on several lists but were told that we'd have to wait 18 months unless we could do our own recruiting. Still getting used to the idea that I would never be able to have a child that was genetically mine, I put appeals up in shop windows, wrote a few articles and even appeared (with photograph!) in a piece in the *Daily Mail*. I was determined to do all that I could to speed the process up.

In the end, donors came from unexpected quarters. In July 2001 I found myself on a train going to Durham where I had two embryos transferred at a London satellite clinic. My husband had had to fly up two nights before to provide his sperm sample, spending the night in a Newcastle airport hotel. Although the transfer went well, no pregnancy resulted and it was the same in January 2002 when my sister voluntarily put herself forward as an egg donor. Fingers crossed that maybe next time will be different.

as if they are being unfaithful to their partner. No one can tell you how you will or should feel. However, once your child becomes a reality, the majority of couples find it no different from conceiving in the 'normal' way. DC Network founder Olivia Montuschi conceived both her children as a result of sperm donation. In a letter from Olivia to would-be DI mums, she writes, 'My huge sadness at not being able to have HIS baby moved on over the years to become a great sense of fulfilment and completeness with the children we did have. It may not be HIS baby, but parenting is all about recognising your child as an individual. It is a rich and rewarding experience that I would not have missed and continue to enjoy.'

What should I tell my child about his or her origins?

There is no legal obligation to tell your child anything if you don't want to. However, many parents who have children by means of donor assisted conception believe that it is best to be open with the child about how he or she was conceived from an early age. They believe that secrecy breeds a lack of trust and makes it more difficult to build a close, loving relationship with their child or children. If you do decide to tell your child you will need to tailor it to his or her age and stage of development. Donor Conception Network publishes some simple story books for children conceived through egg or sperm donation. Later on, you may want to give more information, and your child may want to know more about the donor.

Can my child obtain information about their genetic parent?

If your child was conceived using donor eggs or sperm in the UK, they will have a legal right to obtain non-identifying information about their genetic parentage from the HFEA register when they are 18. Information may include their physical characteristics (such as hair and eye colour), height, ethnic background and likes and dislikes. In the event that two people conceived with donor assisted sperm or eggs want to have children together, the HFEA can tell them whether they share the same genetic parentage, even though their genetic mother or father cannot be identified. However, in order to get information from the HFEA register, children first have to know that they were conceived using donor gametes – so it is up to you to give them the choice to find out this information.

If your child was conceived using donor eggs or sperm from the US and some European countries, they can have access to more information. This may be one reason why you may consider seeking donor assisted conception abroad.

Are there any age restrictions on donors?
Sperm donors must be aged between 18 and 45 while egg donors must be between 18 and 35. This is because eggs from younger women have a higher success rate and there is a lower risk of the eggs having a chromosomal abnormality such as Down's syndrome.

What medical checks do donors have to go through?
Egg and sperm donors have to undergo thorough screening to make sure that they are physically and mentally healthy. A full medical history will be taken and a number of different tests carried out.

Egg donors
- Blood samples. These will be checked for blood group and rhesus (Rh) positive or negative cystic fibrosis, cytomegalovirus (CMV) and sexually transmitted diseases including syphilis, HIV and hepatitis B and C. The donor's blood will also be checked for rubella (German measles) and for levels of LH and FSH.
- If the donor comes from an ethnic group at risk of sickle cell anaemia or thalassaemia, the blood will be screened for these.
- Ultrasound scan. To check the health of the ovaries.

Sperm donors
- Semen sample. To check for the number and quality of sperm.
- Blood samples. As above (excluding rubella)
- If the donor comes from an ethnic group at risk of sickle cell anaemia or thalassaemia, the blood will be screened for these.

Will the donor be tested for HIV?
All donors are tested for HIV and, if they are found to be positive, their semen or eggs will not be used. Because there can be a three-month gap between being infected with HIV and antibodies appearing in the bloodstream, potential donors will be tested twice. If at the second test, a minimum of 180 days after the first, they are HIV-negative, their sperm or eggs may be used.

How can I be sure that the eggs or sperm don't contain any genetic abnormalities?

Donors have to provide a full medical history and will be asked questions about genetic diseases they may have in their family. Testing will also be carried out for cystic fibrosis, a common genetic abnormality that is only passed on when both partners have the faulty gene. If the cystic fibrosis gene is found, the egg or sperm will therefore only be donated to someone who is not a carrier of the gene.

What if the donor is CMV -positive and I'm CMV -negative?

CMV (cytomegalovirus) is one of the family of herpes viruses and is extremely common. In fact, it's estimated that some 80 per cent of adults have CMV antibodies in their blood (a sign they have been infected at some time). The infection can cause an illness similar to 'flu or glandular fever, although in most cases there are no symptoms. A pregnant woman who contracts CMV can pass it on to her unborn baby which in extremely rare cases can cause brain damage and malformations. If you are CMV-negative, only donated eggs or sperm from a donor who is also CMV-negative will be used.

Are egg and sperm donors recruited by the fertility clinic?

Egg donors are largely recruited by clinics but you will be encouraged to recruit one yourself which will help you move higher up the waiting list. Most sperm donors are recruited by a dozen or so sperm banks around the country and most clinics buy in sperm from these. You may also recruit a donor from your family or friends (see p.133–134).

How long will it take to find an egg donor?

It depends. It can take up to a couple of years and often longer. However, clinic waiting lists often fluctuate: an article in the press or an item on a radio programme or TV can bring in several donors and reduce waiting lists dramatically. Clinics that operate egg-sharing schemes, where someone being treated for IVF agrees to share their eggs in return for free or subsidised treatment, tend to have shorter lists. However, concerns about placing too much pressure on women undergoing IVF means that not all clinics run such schemes.

Is there anything we can do to find an egg donor?

- **Media:** Get an article in a newspaper, magazine, radio or TV programme. Try calling the women's editor of your local paper or sending a story or letter to a magazine.
- **Advertising:** Put an advert in the personal column of the local paper or at your health club, gym or doctor's. Many fertility clinics have postcards and ad layouts that you can use. You will have a reference number, so that when the donor contacts the clinic, you will be identified as the person who recruited them and this will enable you to go to the top of the waiting list.
- **Friends and family:** Try to recruit from your family, friends or workmates. This can be a known or anonymous donation. If a relative or friend donates anonymously to the donor pool, you will again be put at the top of the waiting list.

Why is it so difficult to find egg donors?

The HFEA currently specifies that donors must be no older than 35 and recommends that they are anonymous. In this country, donors are not rewarded for their generosity (they can be paid a maximum of £15 for expenses). Add to this that the process involved in egg donation – superovulation and surgical removal of eggs – is time-consuming and uncomfortable, and it is not hard to see why there is a shortage. This is particularly acute among certain groups, such as black and Asian communities. To address the problem and raise public awareness, the National Gamete Donation Trust (NGDT) was founded as a registered charity in April 1998 (www.ngdt.inuk.com).

What kind of people are egg donors?

Donors are not paid in the UK, so people who choose to donate their eggs usually do so because they want to help someone have a baby who might otherwise not have the chance. They include:

- Volunteers. These may come through appeals in the media or sometimes local egg donation campaigns.
- Women who have completed their families and being sterilised.
- Women undergoing IVF who are in an egg-sharing scheme.
- Relatives/friends who donate their eggs to you on a known basis.
- Relatives/friends who donate eggs anonymously to another fertility patient, allowing you to move up the list.

Should I choose an anonymous donor or find a friend/relative willing to donate an egg?

This is an extremely tricky issue. If you choose a known donor, it may raise difficult emotional issues. Research from the US suggests that egg donation from a sister, cousin or friend can be successful, if all concerned are clear about the implications before going ahead. If using a known donor, consider what the relationship of the donor to the child would be, what this person would be called and where to draw the boundaries of the relationship. Some people who choose a known donor do so because they want their child to get to know their donor as a person. Others do so because waiting lists are so long. Counselling is essential because it is vital to be clear about your motivation and how you will deal with the consequences.

What about using a known sperm donor?

It is less common in the UK to use a known sperm donor than a known egg donor. However, some clinics will accept a couple who have found their own donor. Again, you need to be clear about the implications. Some couples import sperm from America in order to provide their child or children with more information about the donor than is allowable here. Some people inseminate themselves outside the clinic system. If you decide to take this route, it is even more important to establish proper boundaries and relationships.

Should I try to find a donor from abroad?

As donors are more readily available abroad (see p.41) this can cut down the length of waiting time and allow you to have more information about the donor. However, travel costs and payment to the donor can be extremely high and you'll need to check carefully what screening procedures are in place in your chosen country. You will also need to think carefully about what the child might need to know about their genetic parents.

How do I choose the right donor and how can I be sure that the donor's characteristics match mine or my partner's?

It depends what factors you feel are important. Some people just want to be parents and aren't too choosy about the donor as long as the child fits into the family in terms of their general appearance.

Others may be more specific. Clinics usually do their best to match donors to the physical characteristics and blood group of a non-genetic parent and may give you a form to fill in where you state your preference for race, hair colour, build and eye colour.

What is the likelihood of a baby having the same physical characteristics as its genetic parent?

Whatever their genetic background, each person is unique in appearance. Sometimes strong features or physical characteristics are passed down from parent to child. In other cases, it can be difficult to see exactly who a child 'takes after'. If you look around the families you know and try to decide how many have children that resemble their parents, chances are it's about half and half. Generally fitting in is probably more important than exact resemblance.

How much will I be told about the donor?

You'll be told about the donor's physical characteristics. Additional information may be available depending on the policy of the clinic and on how much information the donor has disclosed.

How much does this matter?

Some people feel strongly that they want to know about the donor. Others don't mind too much. As your child grows up there may well be times when you wonder if a particular characteristic or trait is that of his or her genetic parent. It pays to remember that any child, however they were conceived, is a result of both genetic and environmental influences. How you bring your child up, the values you teach them and their own personality will play an enormous part in how they turn out. Above all, your child will be a unique individual who looks and behaves quite simply like him or herself.

What does egg donation involve?

Once all the screening tests have been completed, a treatment plan will be worked out. A 'dummy cycle' may be arranged to enable the doctor to observe how long it is likely to take to stimulate your uterine lining before receiving the embryos. After this, you and the donor will be put on a contraceptive pill to synchronise your cycles, followed by ovulation suppressants (see p.74). You will also be given oestrogen in tablet form in order to prepare your uterus for the transfer. During this time, the donor will stop taking suppressants and be given superovulation drugs. She will be scanned to monitor the size of the follicles and you will be scanned to check whether your womb lining is ready for transfer. Egg collection, sperm collection and fertilisation will then proceed as for conventional IVF and the resulting embryos transferred into your uterus. You will then be given progesterone to help support and maintain the lining of your uterus and hopefully the pregnancy. Extra embryos may be frozen.

How many eggs will be donated? Will they be shared with another recipient?

Because of the shortage of egg donors, they may be shared with another recipient but it depends how many ripe eggs are retrieved. Legally no more than 10 children may be born from the same donor.

What happens if the donor changes her mind?

All donors are free to withdraw their consent to the egg donation at any time before a resulting embryo is transferred. In this case, you will usually be offered eggs from another donor.

Can we have sex during the treatment cycle?

The consultant will usually ask you to abstain from penetrative sex during the donation cycle and until the embryo is transferred, to avoid the remote possiblity that you may be pregnant at the time of the transfer. However, your partner should ejaculate two or three times in the week before providing the sperm to be used for fertilisation to ensure the sperm used is the best possible quality.

What are the legal implications of a child conceived using donor eggs/sperm?

If you are married, any child born to you and your husband will be considered to be a child of the marriage and you will be their legal mother, and your husband their legal father. The same applies to unmarried partners, provided your partner has given his written agreement to the treatment. Your child will have all the legal rights that any other child would have, including the right to inherit your property.

Will treatment be confidential?

Under the Human Fertilisation and Embryology Act, clinics are only allowed to communicate information about IVF treatment to those you specify when completing a treatment consent form. Most clinics prefer it if you let them write directly to your GP (or whoever referred you for treatment). However, you can have all letters sent to you to decide whether you wish to forward them to your GP. If you are being funded by a PCT, the clinic will need to send some details to them, in order to collect payment.

Is donor anonymity likely to change?

Since 2000, the government has been consulting on the issue of how much information should be available to people conceived as a result of sperm or egg donation. The consultation period will end in February 2003, but it may be some time before the results are made known. The general climate of opinion is moving towards a policy of greater openness. Removing anonymity would bring donor offspring legislation in line with legislation on adoption, which allows children the right to identifying information about their genetic parents.

How much will my child be able to discover about his or her genetic parent?

At the time of writing, children conceived after August 1991 are able to establish whether they were born as the result of donor conception by consulting the HFEA register when they are 18, or 16 if they intend to marry at that age. At this point, they will be able to discover non-identifying information about their genetic parent and, if they are planning to marry, whether they are related to their intended partner. It has not yet been decided how much information will be made available but it will vary depending on how much information was provided by the donor at the time of donation.

What about embryo donation?

Embryo donation is not widely available. However, some clinics do offer it in cases where there are male and/or female problems – or where a couple is at high risk of passing on a genetic disorder – that make it difficult or impossible to have a child of their own. The embryos will have been donated by a couple who have been undergoing assisted conception and wish to make any 'left over' frozen embryos available to other couples. In this situation, it's especially important to have counselling to ensure that you are aware of the considerable emotional, ethical and legal implications. Most clinics offering embryo donation have long waiting lists.

SURROGACY

Surrogacy – having another woman bear a child for you – is an emotionally intense and legally complex arrangement. It can require vast amounts of time, money and patience to succeed. However couples are increasingly considering surrogacy as a way of having their family. A recent study carried out by the Family and Child Psychology Research Centre at City University, London, has shown that it can be a highly successful and rewarding process. However, all medical, legal, financial and emotional aspects must be thought through by all parties beforehand. Although there is not the scope in this guide to cover all aspects, the following outlines the major issues.

Why would we consider surrogacy?

If you were born without a uterus, have had a hysterectomy or have a medical condition that would make it dangerous for you to become pregnant and give birth. You may also consider it if you have had recurrent miscarriages, numerous attempts at assisted conception but have been unable to conceive or carry a pregnancy to term, or if you have a history of ectopic pregnancies.

What are the different types of surrogacy?

- **Straight surrogacy, also known as natural, traditional or genetic surrogacy** The surrogate ('host') mother is inseminated with the sperm of the intended father, either by artificial insemination or (more rarely) by having sex with the male partner. The host mother is the genetic mother of the child, while the intended father is the genetic father. It is usually arranged by private agreement without the involvement of a fertility clinic, unless donated sperm is used. First you need to find a woman who is prepared to act as a surrogate. It is illegal for a host mother to be paid for offering surrogacy, so she will need to be someone who wants to help you for reasons other than financial gain.

- **Host surrogacy, also known as IVF/GIFT surrogacy, gestational surrogacy, womb leasing** The 'host' mother carries a baby after IVF or GIFT using sperm and eggs from the intended parents of the child. The child is the genetic child of the commissioning couple and has no genetic relationship to the 'host' mother.
- **Gestational surrogacy using a donor egg** This is a variation of IVF surrogacy in which a donor egg is fertilised by the sperm of the intended father. The surrogate mother is again the 'host' mother, or she may be referred to as the 'gestational carrier'. IVF surrogacy can only take place in a clinic licensed by the HFEA for IVF. In this case, the rules are the same as for donated eggs, ie the host mother must be under 35.

Can I find a surrogate through fertility clinics?

Fertility clinics are not allowed to recruit surrogate mothers so it will be up to you to find one. COTS (Childlessness Overcome Through Surrogacy – see p.265) can help and support you through the process.

How do we choose the right surrogate?

You will want to choose someone who is fit and healthy both mentally and physically, and is potentially capable of having a safe healthy pregnancy and birth. It is vital that you trust the surrogate, share the same outlook and goals and all agree on key issues such as prenatal testing and termination for abnormality. Counselling is recommend to help you think about all the issues involved and to ensure that everyone knows where they stand. It is also advisable to seek legal advice and to think about whether you need to take out insurance to cover unanticipated complications.

If we have a surrogate baby, will we have to adopt him or her?

Surrogacy raises some tricky legal issues. The child can be registered in the biological father's surname on its birth certificate. The surrogate mother must be registered as the mother. If she is married, her husband's name will have to go on the certificate, although the baby's surname can be the same as that of its biological parent. There are several options:

- **Parental Responsibility Agreement** The biological father and surrogate can enter into a Parental Responsibility Agreement, sharing equal rights, duties and responsibility for the child. If the surrogate doesn't enter into this, the father can apply for a parental Responsibility Order, which confers these rights on him.

- **Parental Order** If you and the surrogate are in agreement, you and your partner can apply for a Parental Order through the courts, removing the parental rights of the surrogate and transfering them to you. The host mother will have to give up all rights to the child she has carried and by law, she has a right to change her mind about this. It is therefore essential that there is complete trust between you and the host mother.
- **Adoption** If you are married, you can apply for an Adoption Order any time after the baby has been with you for three months. The surrogate mother doesn't have to agree to this.
- **Residence Order** The court can make a Residence Order specifying where the child will live. However, this is not permanent.

What other factors should I take into consideration?
- Do you feel you are emotionally strong enough to cope with the stress of using a surrogate?
- What support will you have from family and friends?
- What is the motivation of the surrogate mother?
- How much support will be available to her as she goes through pregnancy and birth and handing over the baby to you?
- How do you feel about another woman becoming pregnant with your partner's sperm after so many years of difficult and expensive treatment has failed to help you to become pregnant?
- How much contact will you have with the surrogate during her pregnancy? COTS recommends that you should keep in regular contact with the surrogate and visit her on a regular basis.
- What expenses will you provide eg maternity clothes?
- How do you feel about pre-natal testing?
- How do you feel about having to adopt the baby?
- Will you maintain links with the surrogate?
- What will you tell your child about its origins?
- How would you feel if the surrogate decides she doesn't want to hand over the baby?

Adoption

Adoption is intended to give children who, for whatever reason, cannot live in their birth family, the chance to have a happy, secure life in another family. Legally, it involves transferring the care of the child and all the parental rights and responsibilities from his or her birth parent(s) to you by means of an Adoption Order. The process of adoption differs from fertility treatment in that the emphasis shifts from fulfilling your desire for a child onto the needs of a child for parents and a secure family background.

Adoption is likely to work best if you are able to put the heartbreak of infertility behind you and embrace it as a positive choice to give a child a new start in life. For this reason, most agencies will not usually take you on until six months to a year after completing fertility treatment, to ensure that you have come to terms with all the issues surrounding your fertility problems.

Although there is not enough scope in this guide to cover every aspect of adoption, the following covers the major issues involved.

How do we go about adopting?

The majority of adoptions in the UK are done through local authority social services departments (approximately 200) or through voluntary adoption agencies (approximately 37). Although it does not directly place children for adoption, or approve prospective adoptive parents, the British Association for Adoption and Fostering (BAAF) has a database of fostering and adoption agencies on its website: baaf.org.uk. You can also find information and a list of adoption agencies in the BAAF's book *Adopting a Child, An essential guide for anyone taking their first steps towards adopting a child in the UK* by Jenifer Lord.

What will we need to do in the first instance?

You will need to contact agencies covering your area. They will usually send you general information and arrange an informal meeting so that you can decide whether you want to proceed. You can contact a number of agencies at this stage, although you can only follow through with one.

What should we do if the agency won't take us on?

It is rare to be turned down once you have gone through the preparation period (see below) but some people do get turned down by an agency right at the beginning of the process. If you do not meet the needs of one agency, you may be more successful with another. It may be that you don't quite fit their criteria straightaway or because you have only just finished fertility treatment the agency will suggest that you contact them again in a year or so. If you do get turned down, don't despair that you will never adopt. Take some time to think about why you were not successful and look for another agency.

If we're taken on by an agency, how can we prepare ourselves?

Virtually all agencies run preparation courses designed to help prospective parents and Adoption UK (www.adoptionuk.org.uk and helpline 0870 7700 450) has a range of materials for those looking into adopting. Some of the issues you might think about are:

- What will you tell your child about being adopted?
- How might you help your child feel a sense of identity with his or her birth family and culture?
- How would you feel about maintaining some sort of contact with your child's birth parents?
- What is your attitude towards your child wanting to trace his or her birth parents?

What happens next?

When you have attended the preparation group, the social worker will visit you at home a number of times to make a full assessment of you and any other members of your household. A report on you will be prepared and put before an adoption panel, consisting of social workers, other professionals, independent people with experience of adoption and people employed by the adoption agency. They have the authority to decide whether a child should be made available for adoption, whether you should be approved and whether you are suitable for a particular child or children. The report is designed to establish that you will be able to care for the child and cater for his or her needs into young adulthood and will include:

- personal details including your age, your education, job, income and details of relationship.

- your living conditions, home environment and neighbourhood.
- how you feel about your infertility.
- your views about upbringing and discipline.
- your health, fitness and emotional well-being.
- whether you have a health problem or any unhealthy habits.
- your ethnic background and culture.
- your language.
- your religion, if any.
- your relationships with family and friends, and the kind of support available to you.
- how well the social worker considers you will be able to meet the needs of the child as it grows up.

Will there be any formal checks?

As well as assessing your suitability and your reasons for wanting to adopt a child, the agency will need to perform some formal checks. These include:

- Criminal record check on you and any other adults living in your household. You will have to give written permission for this.
- Local authority check.
- Personal references.
- Full medical report.

What will happen after we've been approved by the adoption panel. Will we be able to adopt a child straightaway?

At this stage only around 5 per cent of those applying to adopt are turned down. You will be placed on a waiting list for a child. Once one has been found and has lived with your for at least three months, you can apply to the court for an Adoption Order to remove parental rights and responsibilities from the child's birth parents and transfer them to both of you (if you are married) or you as a single parent. Once the order has been made, the child will become a full member of your family and have exactly the same rights and privileges as if it were your birth child.

Does it matter if I'm not married?

Single people are eligible to adopt. If you are living with a partner but are not married, you won't be able to adopt jointly as only

Liza Lorenz, 37

I had lymphatic cancer when I was 17 but wasn't warned that the treatment might make me infertile, although afterwards I suspected it had. When we got married, my husband and I tried for a baby for a while without success so I went to the GP. I had been getting hot flushes and the GP referred me to a specialist at the local hospital. I was diagnosed with premature menopause and put on HRT. Although I was producing eggs, they weren't of good enough quality to be fertilised. This meant that egg donation was my only chance of having a baby. We decided we would give it two or three attempts and, if it failed, to go for adoption.

We chose a large private hospital in London and I had to wait two years to find a donor who matched the right physical characteristics (eye colour, height etc). I had three eggs transferred but didn't become pregnant. I was devastated but we decided we would try again. Unfortunately, I didn't conceive the next time either. That really knocked me and I was probably at my lowest point. I found it very hard to tell my husband that IVF had failed again.

I realised that I really had had enough of IVF so we decided to apply for adoption. I'd always said I wanted two children and that even if we had a baby by IVF I would like to adopt a child.

At first we applied to a local borough council but they said that at 36 and 37 respectively, we were too old. Eventually we applied to a voluntary agency which we found through friends who had adopted through them. It took us three years in all: over a year to be approved and a long time to get the home study done and another four months for the report to be written because the social worker was so overworked. The whole process was incredibly draining.

Eventually we were approved and we now have two lovely children, a brother and sister aged 11 months and 21 months. I feel so lucky to have a baby, first because we never thought we would have one and also because I was quite prepared to adopt older children.

The experience of infertility has brought us closer as a couple. I was very disillusioned with the hospital where we had our IVF. It was like a factory: completely impersonal. I received no useful counselling and was not even told I could have a free follow-up consultation following the failure of the egg donation.

In all we spent £10,000, which we took from our savings. I now regret spending so much money on IVF that we could have spent on the children. My advice to other people would be to shop around for a clinic and not be taken in by smooth-talking doctors. Most private hospitals are only interested in your money and their success rate, not you as a person. You should also decide at the outset how many times you will try IVF – it is very easy to keep trying and not look at other options.

married couples can do this. In this case, one of you can adopt and your partner can apply for a residence order, which confers responsibility for the child until he or she is 16 or, exceptionally, 18.

What are the chances of being able to adopt a baby?

Most children placed for adoption are older. According to BAAF, the number of healthy white babies placed for adoption under a year old is on average one or less per local authority per year, although 59 per cent of children adopted are aged between one and four years.

What information will the agency give us about the child?

Relevant background knowledge about the child you are planning to adopt will help you care for them in a way that is sensitive to their needs. The agency is legally obliged to give you this information which should include:

- Details about your child's background.
- If they have been in care, number of placements and how long they lasted.
- Education and progress at school.
- Medical information.

How long is it likely to take?

This can vary a lot. The average length of time from being assessed to the adoption order being passed currently stands at just over two years. The Government's Adoption Standards document gives details of recommended timescales. Adoption legislation is currently being overhauled and a new Adoption and Children Bill should be in place by 2004. You can find more information on the Government's website: www.doh.gov.uk/adoption.

What kind of support can we get after we have adopted?

Many adoption agencies provide post-adoption support. Adoption UK also offers information, advice and encouragement (see above).

What can my child find out about their birth parents?

Adopted children have the right to see their birth certificate at the age of 18. Many adopters exchange a letter with the child's birth parents with news of the child via the adoption agency once a year.

The National Organisation for Counselling Adoptees and Parents (NORCAP) offers help and advice to adult children who wish to trace their birth parents (www.norcap.org.uk, tel 01865 87500).

Should we consider adopting a child from abroad?

If you are unable to adopt in the UK, or if you feel you would be unable to care for an older child, you may consider adopting a child from another country. You will have to be approved by your local authority to do this and undergo all the same checks as if you were adopting a child in the UK. Adopting a child from overseas can be costly, time-consuming and stressful, as you need to consider a number of different emotional, social and practical issues, eg how will you enable an adopted child to adjust to a new life here, whilst keeping a sense of their cultural identity.

How much is it likely to cost?

It can cost anything from £5000 to £25,000, including the cost of a home assessment, plus travelling, accommodation, charges for local legal advice, documents and certificates.

How do we go about it?

In the first instance, discuss your intentions with your local authority adoption agency. Also contact the embassy of the country from which you wish to adopt. You can get more information from www.doh.gov.uk/adoption/intercountry/faq. Help, advice and support is available from the Overseas Adoption Helpline's Advice Line on 0870 516 8742 or www.oah.org.uk/adviceline.

Should we consider fostering and, if so, how should we go about it?

If you can't or don't want to adopt, fostering can be a way to help a child who is unable to be cared for in their own home until they are either able to return home or until they reach adulthood. If you are interested you should approach your local social services or social work department, or an independent fostering agency. You can get information from the BAAF and from the Fostering Network (www.thefostering.net).

Coping with fertility problems

It is extremely common to feel strong emotions as you go through the process of discovering you have fertility problems and then undergoing all the different investigations and treatments.

Infertility can be viewed as a form of bereavement that calls into question everything you ever hoped for or expected from your life. Like any other bereavement, it can produce almost unbearable feelings of loss and longing. Having children may have been something you always planned to do and now you are being asked to give up your dreams of having a child easily and 'naturally'.

You may feel your body has let you down in the most fundamental way. If you have been used to planning your life, you may feel a devastating sense of loss of control. Not only that but the whole of your life now seems to revolve around what you fear may be an impossible task.

There is not necessarily a smooth progression through these different emotions. Your feelings may ebb and flow at different times. Sometimes they may feel perfectly manageable, at others they may become overwhelming. The following are some common reactions but they are by no means the only ones.

- When you first learn that you have fertility problems, you may feel shock, disbelief and deep disappointment, or that it isn't really happening to you and that you will wake up one morning and find it isn't really true.

- A period of acute grief may follow as you accept the diagnosis and try to come to terms with it. It may be hard to eat, sleep or concentrate.

- You may experience anger. You may blame yourself, or your partner for your situation or feel guilty that something you have done is responsible for your infertility. You may regret putting off having a family or if your partner didn't want children earlier, you may wish you'd got pregnant 'by accident'.

- You may be jealous of people who do have children, or find it unbearable to be around families and feel cut off or deliberately isolate yourself from your family and friends.

- As treatment begins you may be full of hope, only to plummet to the depths of despair if it doesn't work.

- Some people keep on trying IVF again and again, even though their chances of success are dwindling. Each disappointment may be followed by a renewed hope that 'maybe next time it will work'.

- One of the hardest things to bear is often the uncertainty: will you eventually become pregnant and if you do, will you have a baby? Or will all your efforts come to nothing? No matter what treatment you try or how much money you can afford to pay, no one can offer you any guarantees.

How can I cope with all these different feelings?

Fertility treatment is a roller coaster and there is no right or wrong way to deal with your feelings. It is a question of trial and error and finding what works best for you.

- **Try to stick to your usual routine** Going to work, taking regular exercise, eating well, getting enough sleep and making time to do things that you enjoy may help to keep emotions on an even keel.

- **Work out how much information you can cope with** Some couples find having as much information as possible to be the best way to feel more in control. You could buy books, collect leaflets and look on the Internet – some of the US sites such as RESOLVE (www.resolve.org) have excellent material. If knowing too much makes you more anxious, then inform yourself as much as you need to, but don't become obsessed with information gathering, and don't feel guilty if there are some areas you don't know about.

- **Try a complementary therapy** Yoga, meditation or relaxation-based treatment may help you to deal with stress and relax.

- **Learn to manage stress** A book on stress management, using a relaxation tape or attending a stress management course may be useful. ISSUE has a fact sheet on stress and can also provide details of stress management courses.

- **Consider ways to make life easier for yourself** If your work or life is already extremely stressful, the pressure of fertility treatment can be the final straw, and little things can start to get you down. You may want to consider taking a less demanding job or getting help with things you have to do at home.

- **Take some time out** Schedule time to do things just for you, such as making time to exercise, a soak in a warm bath, a massage or weekend away.
- **Get support** Sharing feelings usually makes them easier to manage. If you feel that you can't talk to your family and friends – or even if you can – you may find that talking things over with someone who has been through the same experience themselves brings a tremendous sense of comfort and relief. There are some excellent support groups (see p.265), some of which have local groups and/or sub-groups specialising in particular issues.
- **Talk it over** Many couples find that counselling is invaluable. It is considered to be so important that every licensed fertility treatment centre in the UK has to provide it by law. Talking to someone who understands your feelings, but is not directly involved, can give you a sense of perspective. You may dislike the idea of counselling and feel that you should be able to cope alone, or that the counsellor will judge you in some way or tell you what to do. You may even fear, especially if your situation is an unconventional one, that the counsellor will stop you from having treatment. These fears, although perfectly natural, are almost certainly unfounded. No properly trained counsellor will either judge you or tell you what you should be doing or try to stop you from doing what you want. Rather they will help you to talk through your feelings and enable you to focus on finding your own solutions.

Will counselling be provided by the clinic?

All clinics are obliged to offer you counselling if your treatment involves assisted conception or gamete donation but the amount provided varies a great deal. Some clinics offer unlimited sessions, others may only offer a set number of free sessions, after which you would have to pay to see the counsellor. There are three broad types of counselling:

- **Implications counselling** This is the mandatory counselling designed to ensure that you understand exactly what treatment is being offered, why it is being offered and its implications. It will be offered by a consultant or a dedicated counsellor, and is free of charge.

- **Support counselling** Fertility treatment is notoriously stressful. Support counselling may be provided by a qualified counsellor but other members of staff – such as specialist fertility nurses – are also trained to take on this role in some clinics. However, you may feel more comfortable talking to a counsellor who is completely independent of your treatment. Many clinics offer independent counsellors, others don't.
- **Therapeutic counselling** Infertility can often raise issues in your life generally. Therapeutic counselling is intended to address these and to help you think about the consequences of your treatment and be realistic in your expectations. You may be charged extra for this type of counselling at the clinic. Alternatively, you may be referred to an independent counsellor whom you will have to pay yourself.

What might happen at my counselling session?

This will largely depend on the type of counselling and its purpose, the approach of the counsellor and your needs. At implications counselling you will usually be offered factual information to help you to understand exactly what a treatment or decision involves and enable you to make decisions. Support counselling may happen as you are actually undergoing treatment rather than in a dedicated session. Ideally, a therapeutic counselling session should provide you with the opportunity to clarify your situation and the issues you face and explore your feelings about them. The counsellor's role is to offer a non-judgemental sounding board in order to enable you to explore all these things freely without fear of criticism or judgement. The counsellor should not give you direct advice but should encourage you (and your partner) to find your own solutions. Anything you say to the counsellor will be confidential.

Can we attend counselling sessions together?

Infertility is a problem involving couples, so it is preferable to attend implications counselling sessions together. It is up to you and your partner to decide whether you attend therapeutic counselling together, separately or a mixture of the two.

Sabeha Syed, 38

I've always had irregular periods. In fact, when I was 15, I went for a year and a half without menstruating and at 21 I was diagnosed with polycystic ovary syndrome. I knew then that I might have problems with having a baby but, as I didn't particularly want children at that stage, it wasn't a priority.

When I was 33, my husband and I decided we would like a child. I was aware it might be difficult (if not impossible) to conceive. I also knew that fertility treatment could take time, so we only tried for a few months before seeking help. I've been at the same endocrinology unit since I was 21 and was referred to their reproductive medicine clinic, whose attitude was 'let's not waste time'. I had all my treatment under the NHS.

I had diathermy, where they zap the follicles in an attempt to stimulate ovulation. That seemed to regulate my periods to about every six weeks or so. The consultant gave me a window of around six months to a year at the most in which to get pregnant, after which she said she would put me on Clomid.

Six months went by and I had made an appointment to start on Clomid when I discovered I was pregnant. Unfortunately I lost the baby at eight weeks. I had to wait another few months before starting on Clomid.

In July 1999 I took Clomid for five days and had to go back to see how the follicles were developing. One follicle looked promising so they gave me an hCG injection to stimulate ovulation and told me to go home and have sex for four days! It may sound like fun, but in fact it was enormously stressful, so much so that when I went back for my appointment I told them that if it hadn't worked I would go for artificial insemination next time! However, I was lucky. It worked first time and I gave birth to Louis in April 2000.

I am now planning to have another baby, but since I had Louis I have developed an underactive thyroid. I am aware that this, combined with my age (I'm now 38) and the PCOS, makes it likely that I will have further problems. I'm fairly philosophical about the whole thing. I'm an only child so I don't think it's the worst thing in the world. I've just had all the blood tests done and I am due to go back next week for the results. On the plus side, I am having a regular cycle now, although I don't know if I am ovulating. If they advise Clomid, I will go for it again but I wouldn't have IVF. I've seen too many people go through it, and I wouldn't want to go down that road.

I think it is important to keep fertility treatment in the open and talk to people. You need all the support you can get, especially if the worst happens and you miscarry. Fortunately, because everyone knew about my treatment they were all very supportive when I had my miscarriage. It is also vital to be kind to yourself. If you can't bear to be around children, don't force yourself. I didn't have a problem being around children, but I couldn't bear to be near pregnant women. It wasn't that I wanted their children, but I wanted so much to be pregnant myself.

Subfertility is like a bereavement and it's possible to become very obsessed and have this idealised child in your mind. When you see people with children you think, 'These people have everything.' I now realise that this is not the case. Even though I've been lucky, I do think it's important not to lose sight of what else you have in your life.

Is my partner likely to feel the same way as me?

Every one faced with fertility problems will have his or her own unique feelings and ways of dealing with them. How your partner feels is likely to depend on his perception of the problem – how important having a family is to him, whether he feels less of a man or that it is his fault. It is often the case that there is a difference in the type of feelings that men and women feel most comfortable with and how they express them. Men may feel it easier to express anger rather than grief, or throw themselves into work or a hobby rather than weep, and often adopt a more 'problem-solving' approach to emotional difficulties than women. As infertility isn't a problem that can be easily solved, this can lead to feelings of frustration and anger.

It is important to recognise that your partner will not necessarily respond in the way that you might expect. The main thing is to try to keep the lines of communication open between you, to share how you are each feeling and try to understand and respect any differences.

What effect can fertility treatment have on my relationship?

The stress of fertility treatment can affect the dynamics between you and may change your relationship. Some couples feel they are drawn closer together by the experience, others find that they respond very differently and it can drive a wedge between them.

If you've planned for a family, either or both of you may feel you are letting your partner down. All joy and spontaneity can be lost and it can sometimes seem as if your life has contracted down to nothing but the making of a baby.

- Decide between you how long you will carry on with fertility treatment, how much you will spend and when you will stop.
- Consider taking a treatment break or a holiday if the stress of treatment is becoming too much.
- Make time to be together and to do things you enjoy as a couple, not as a couple trying for a baby.
- Some couples find it helps to set limits on the time they will talk about it eg no more than an hour a day.
- Try to avoid blame – either self-blame or of each other.
- Share your feelings honestly, even if they are different.
- Accept what your partner is feeling, even if he is feeling different things at different times to you.

- You may want to ration the number of baby-related activities you attend eg christenings, without becoming isolated.
- Think about joining a support group (see p.157 and p.265).

We are finding scheduled sex very hard to cope with. Is there anything we can do?

Couples with fertility problems often say that their sex life suffers when they have to have sex on demand. Having sex becomes about making a baby rather than having fun and showing your desire and love for each other. This can lead to other problems, such as failure to have an erection, or vaginismus. On top of this, it can be hard to feel desirable when your body is pumped full of hormones and your most basic physical functions are subject to investigation and analysis.

Psychologists who are experienced in dealing with couples undergoing fertility treatment often advise them to focus on having sex during non-fertile times of the month, purely for the enjoyment of it. Massage is a great relaxer and can be a another way to be physically intimate with your partner. Touching and showing your affection in other ways is important. If you feel that sexual problems are affecting your relationship, counselling or help from a relationship counsellor can help you get back on track.

What should we tell our family and friends?

Many couples find the issue of what and whether to tell family and friends about their difficulties one of the hardest to handle. You may feel that those around you will not be sympathetic or that they cannot possibly understand what you are going through and the way you are feeling. If you do tell people, it can sometimes feel that your private life is an open book and you may dislike the fact that people feel entitled to comment on the most personal aspects of it.

- Think about who you will tell and what you will tell them. You may find that those you talk to are sensitive to your feelings and make a real effort to understand. Equally, some of those closest to you aren't terribly sympathetic or make tactless remarks, perhaps in an attempt to be helpful.
- Let people know how they can help you. Many people are insensitive because they simply don't know much about fertility problems, so arm yourself with facts to correct any

misconceptions and help other people to help you. You may
want to tell those close to you exactly how they can best support
you, eg, calling you after a test or treatment or perhaps waiting
until you are ready to tell them.

- Prepare for insensitive questions such as 'Don't you want to have
  a family then?' Your counsellor or members of your support group
  will be able to give you plenty of ideas as to how to answer them.

I've had several failed attempts at IVF. I feel devastated – would it help to take a break from treatment?

Taking a break can often help you regain some perspective and
decide how you want to proceed. You may want to take a
geographical break by putting some distance between you and your
infertility problems. You could also take some time for yourself eg
booking a beauty treatment, reading a book or meeting up with
people you like and have fun with. If, having taken a break, you still
feel you aren't coping well, it is worth considering seeking further
help from your doctor. You may be becoming depressed (see below).

I can't seem to escape my feelings of unhappiness. Should I seek professional help?

Sometimes the feelings brought up by the experience of fertility
problems and treatment can be so overwhelming that you are
unable to deal with them. Infertility is recognised as a life-crisis
and, as such, it can sometimes trigger other painful memories or
unresolved issues from the past. It can be hard to recognise when
your feelings are part of the normal process that most people with
fertility problems go through, or when they indicate a deeper
problem such as depression. This can lead to persistent low mood
and tearfulness that you can't seem to shift, irritability, anxiety and
insomnia. It can also bring about a loss of appetite or weight, lack of
energy and stamina, loss of interest in sex as well as low self-esteem,
and feelings of guilt and helplessness.

How would I cope with remaining childless?

At some point, you may have to face up to the fact that you will
never have children. Everyone who comes to this point has to cope
in their own way and at their own pace. After a period of mourning

their childlessness, some couples feel it is a relief to forget about the quest for a child, especially after many years of stressful treatment. Even then you may suddenly feel devastation at family gatherings, anniversaries of a treatment failure or when you see families in the park. Many psychologists suggest considering the following questions to try to understand these feelings:

- Why did you want a child?
- What kind of things would you be able to do if you had children? How might you be able to do them without children?
- What kind of things will you be able to do without children?
- How might your life be better/worse without a child or children?
- What kind of things did you enjoy doing before you started the quest to have a child? Would you still want to do these things?
- What other things do you want to do with your life apart from having children? How might you go about achieving these?

A childfree life can bring many different rewards – more time to spend with friends and relatives, more energy to develop your career or to devote to other interests, skills or talents. You may choose to find a way of being involved with children, eg by playing a part in the lives of nephews and nieces. Many couples find it helps mark the end of one phase of their life (trying for a child) and the beginning of their future. These can include taking a holiday or holding a personal or public ritual of some kind. Above all, bear in mind that a life free of children – even unwillingly – can be just as enjoyable, fulfilling, creative and rewarding as one with children.

Are there support groups?
MoreToLife (see p.266) is a support group set up by ISSUE to help those who are exploring all that a life without children has to offer, whether or not they are still undergoing fertility treatment or have never had it. The group aims to promote a positive outlook, while accepting the need for people to grieve and have support in adjusting to this new phase of their lives.

MoreToLife has a range of fact sheets, including Living without Children, Coping Strategies, Contact with Children, Stopping Treatment, Men's Issues, Relationships and Family, Friends & Colleagues, and also holds workshops which many couples find extremely helpful.

Clinics and Specialists

Costs and funding

Who can get treatment on the NHS?

Theoretically, NHS treatment is free to all who need it. In practice, whether or not you will get fertility treatment depends on a host of criteria that vary from one area to another. These include your age, the number of previous children you have had (if any), how long you have been in your relationship and the number of previous treatment cycles. The exact criteria vary tremendously. To give just one example, according to NIAC, the maximum age limit for treatment is 34 in some areas and 43 in others. Some health authorities (HAs) specify that couples must be married. To complicate matters further, most HAs don't apply criteria evenly across the board – according to NIAC, 63 per cent have criteria for IVF but only 19 per cent for tubal surgery.

What restrictions might there be on us getting help through the NHS?

At present, fertility treatment is not considered to be an essential treatment and comes far down on the list of priorities for most local HA budgets. There may be restrictions based on the following:

- Age. Many authorities will only treat women under a certain age.
- Marital status. Some authorities refuse to fund unmarried couples.
- The type of treatment you need. A quarter of authorities do not fund assisted conception treatments like IVF. Even if your health authority does fund treatment, it may not provide the treatment recommended for you. For example, most health authorities will fund ovulation induction (fertility drugs) and tubal surgery but not assisted conception. In some cases this may mean that you are offered a treatment that is not the one you need.
- If your authority does fund IVF, there may be restrictions on the number of treatment cycles it is prepared to fund. This ranges from one to three, depending on where you live.
- Your postcode. NHS treatment is a 'postcode lottery' that depends very largely on where you live.

What will the NHS fund?

The NHS should fund initial investigations carried out by your GP or at your local NHS hospital. You may also be eligible to be funded for some straightforward treatments such as infertility drugs and IUI using your partner's sperm at a local hospital. However, only a quarter of assisted conception treatments are funded by the NHS. If you need more sophisticated assisted conception techniques, such as IVF, and are being treated at a specialist fertility clinic, the NHS will not currently subsidise it directly, because it is not considered to be part of general medical care. You may still be able to get funding if your HA or primary care trust (PCT) has a contract with the clinic at which you are being treated. This may or may not be a clinic in your local area. Some specialised fertility clinics provide drugs on the NHS.

What is the difference between a health authority and a PCT?

Many changes are currently going on in the health service to make it less centralised, more cost-efficient and more responsive to the needs of those on the frontline – patients, doctors, nurses and other staff involved in providing services. The main change has been to give local PCTs responsibility for planning and developing services in their local area. The old HAs, which used to be responsible for the management of health services in different areas of the country, have been abolished and 28 new strategic health authorities (StHAs) created, each serving around 1.5 million people. They act as a parent body and provide a link between the department of health (DOH) and the NHS in each area, supporting PCTs and Trusts in delivering the government's NHS Plan. A map of StHAs can be seen at www.doh.gov.uk/shiftingthebalance/haconsultation/sthamap.htm. Contact details for your local PCT can also be found on the internet at www.doh.gov.uk/pricare/pdfs/pctcontactsjuly02.pdf. The National Institute for Clinical Excellence (NICE), set up to advise the government on the efficacy and cost-effectiveness of treatments, is trying to iron out anomalies in the provision of infertility treatment by compiling new guidelines for England and Wales (Scotland already has guidelines). In future, this may mean that fertility treatment will be funded and delivered on a much more equitable basis throughout the country, although there are still likely to be restrictions on who is eligible for funding.

How do I find out if I am likely to get funding?

In this section, we tell you what treatments each clinic provides on the NHS. In addition, your GP, the clinic where you are being treated and/or one of the fertility support groups may know what the situation is in your area. Alternatively, you can get information from NIAC's Annual Survey of NHS Funding of Infertility Services. This has up-to-date details on which treatments are available on the NHS in different areas. Bear in mind that even if you are eligible for funding, there is likely to be a waiting list.

Can I appeal if I'm refused funding?

You can, but if the PCT doesn't provide funding, you need to be prepared for your appeal to be unsuccessful. You should also consider the time an appeal could potentially take. Rather than appealing individually, you may want to get involved in NIAC's campaign for a central policy for funding across the country. NIAC suggests writing to your MP and to the chief executive of the local PCT and asking them to review their policy. NIAC suggests that when writing you include the following points:

- Ask the PCT to justify current policy and request a review.
- Emphasise that infertility is a health problem and, as such, should be funded.
- Explain what effect lack of provision is having on you and other couples you know with fertility problems.
- Ask your GP what the demand for treatment is in your district and let the PCT know that it is failing to meet the needs of people requiring treatment.
- Don't be put off. If you don't succeed, try again!

Can I pay for my own treatment at an NHS unit?

If the PCT won't fund your treatment or you don't want to wait until funds are available, you can often choose to 'self-fund'. This means that the clinic will charge you a similar price for treatment as it charges the PCT. It is different from private treatment, as you will receive exactly the same care as people funded by the PCT. The charges are non-profit-making (unlike private treatment) and cover the cost of staff and equipment plus investigations. All income goes back into the NHS rather than to a private company.

How much is private fertility treatment likely to cost?

This will depend on exactly what treatments you are having, how many you have and how you are planning to fund treatment – that is whether you will be getting some treatment on the NHS, will be self-funding or going completely for private treatment. One thing is certain, fertility treatment can often run into tens of thousands of pounds and the more high-tech the treatment, the higher the cost. Some couples sell or remortgage their houses to pay for treatment.

What will the costs be made up of?

In this section, we tell you how much each clinic charges for their services. Costs will consist of a combination of the following:

- Consultation fees. The first consultation is usually longer and costs more but you will also have to budget for subsequent consultations, which is why it's important to find out how many times you are likely to need to see the consultant.
- Routine investigations eg hormone blood tests, two–five day ultrasound scan, semen analysis and vaginal swabs.
- Further specialist investigations eg hysterosalpingogram, follicle tracking, ovarian cyst aspiration, trial embryo transfer, chromosome analysis, cystic fibrosis screen and antiphospholipid screening (if you have recurrent miscarriage).
- Fertility drugs.
- Treatment eg IUI, DI, IVF, ICSI, FET, ovum donation with IVF/ICSI, blastocyst culture-assisted hatching, frozen embryo donation.
- Embryo/semen freezing and storage fees.
- HFEA fee (see below).

To help compare clinics, ask if they can send you a price list, whether they have any 'package deals' and be aware of any additional costs you may have to pay (eg consultations, embryo storage etc). Also check whether you will be eligible for a refund if a treatment cycle has to be abandoned. Some clinics accept the results of tests carried out elsewhere so you will not have to pay for them to be repeated – check which ones these are.

What is the HFEA fee and will I have to pay it?

The HFEA charges a licence fee per IVF/frozen embryo replacement cycle and for donor assisted conception. Currently these stand at £36 and £14 respectively. Sometimes this fee will be shown separately or it will be included in the overall 'package'.

Will I have to pay for each treatment separately?
For consultation and tests, you will usually be asked to pay in full on the day the test is carried out. For treatment cycles, including drugs, tests and monitoring, you may be asked to pay in advance – often on the first day of monitoring for each treatment cycle.

Will I have to pay for my own drugs?
It depends whether your local PCT agrees to fund some or all of them. If your PCT won't pay, you will have to buy them yourself – either through the hospital pharmacy or through one of the schemes detailed below. If you are being treated in an NHS hospital and buy drugs through their pharmacy, you will usually pay the NHS cost plus possibly a small extra charge. Some private clinics insist that you buy drugs from their pharmacy.

Is there any way I can get the drugs more cheaply?
If you can, it is worth shopping around for fertility drugs as prices can vary enormously. Three drug companies – Ferring, Organon and Serono – offer Home Care schemes in which all the drugs and equipment you need (eg syringes, swabs and instructions) are delivered direct to your home at a convenient time. They also provide telephone back-up. Ask the fertility clinic about the various schemes. Once you have your prescription, you'll need to register for the scheme before the drugs can be delivered. The drug companies have separate contracts with different fertility clinics based on how many drugs the clinic prescribes, so prices will vary depending on where you are being treated. The larger the fertility clinic and the more treatment cycles they perform, the less the drugs are likely to cost. You should be aware that some clinics charge a handling fee for issuing your prescription and contacting Home Care on your behalf.

What other costs are involved in my treatment?
You will have to budget for travel and parking fees if the clinic is not close to home. You might also have to allow for any unscheduled time off work that you may need whilst undergoing treatment.

How much do fees vary between different private clinics?

To be competitive, most private clinics have similar costs. It can be difficult to compare them directly because of the way these are split – some list each treatment separately, others as a package. The best way to find out is to get a few price lists, sit down with a calculator and work it out.

What is a payment plan?

Some clinics have payment plans designed to help you spread the cost of drugs and treatment. Some offer package deals eg a single-cycle package that includes consultation, scan and drugs, or a three-cycle package for a set price. These allow you to obtain treatment at a lower cost than if you paid for each cycle separately. Of course, the disadvantage is that if you do become pregnant on the first or second treatment cycle you won't get your money back for the third.

How much will I have to pay if the treatment is cancelled?

It depends. In some clinics, if treatment is cancelled for medical reasons (eg poor response to drugs) you will only be charged for scans and administration. If, however, you decide to cancel for other reasons, you may well be charged the full cost of the whole cycle.

Is fertility treatment covered by insurance?

Some private health insurance plans will cover the cost of the initial consultation and tests, although treatment is not usually covered. FertilityConfidential (www.fertilityconfidential.com) has a list of the major UK health insurers and their policy on funding for tests. Alternatively, call your insurance company. A new insurer, IRMS (tel 01284 747090 or ivf@irms.co.uk), will refund IVF costs should you miscarry after treatment (the miscarriage must occur after a positive pregnancy scan, usually 60 days after treatment). Although losing your unborn baby is probably not something you want to think about, the policy does at least mean that you won't be prevented by financial considerations from trying again if you want to.

I really can't afford the treatment. What can I do?

- Friends and/or relatives may be willing to lend or give you the money. Money is a very sensitive issue in personal relationships, so if you do decide to approach someone you know, it is important to establish whether you are being offered a loan or a gift, and if it is a loan, to make arrangements to pay whoever it is back.

- You may be able to get a bank loan or a credit card with a low APR. BMI Healthcare has a credit card that can be used for medical treatment at any of the BMI centres with a fertility unit. The card offers six months interest-free credit with a minimum monthly payment of 5 per cent of the balance or £25, whichever is larger. If you can pay off the whole balance within six months, there is no extra charge. Ask your fertility unit whether it has the card.

- You may want to consider moving to another area in an effort to get funding on the NHS. Before you take this drastic step, you will need up-to-date information on which HAs or PCTs fund treatment, together with details of their eligibility criteria and waiting lists. Some HAs that previously funded treatment have now closed their lists, although they will still honour their existing agreements. FertilityConfidential has a list on its website or contact one of the other infertility organisations.

- FertilityConfidential (www.fertilityconfidential.com) is planning to set up a charity to provide funds for IVF and ICSI for couples who really cannot afford it. To be eligible, you must be UK residents, registered with a GP for at least 12 months and have no living children within the relationship. You'll need a letter from your GP and the medical director of the clinic confirming that you need fertility treatment.

- Consider becoming a resident of another EU country that is known to have Government funding for fertility treatment. Reciprocal arrangements within the EU entitles you to the same medical treatment as their residents.

I've heard that if I donate eggs (ie join an egg-sharing scheme) I could get my treatment costs reduced. Is this true?

In order to cut waiting lists for egg donation, some clinics have introduced shared egg schemes in which you agree to donate half of any eggs recovered through IVF to another couple having fertility treatment. This means that if you produce ten eggs, you will give five away. In return, the woman using your eggs will pay for part of your treatment.

How to use the funding table

This shows the types of treatments funded by the NHS across the UK, where this information has been provided. Please note that information was requested from health authorities (HAs) at the time when primary care trusts (PCTs) took over responsibility for services such as fertility treatment. Many PCTs have carried over the existing health authority policy as an interim measure, whilst others will have formulated their own policy on funding as soon as they came into existence. For this reason, information returned by HAs still appears in the table, even though they have now been replaced by one or more PCT. If funding details for your local area are not listed in the table, you should contact your local PCT for information (see p.161).

Upper age limits can relate to maximum age at time of GP referral or at start of treatment. They may not relate to all treatments funded – if this is the case, they usually apply to IVF/ICSI. Criteria relating to existing children from current or past relationships can indicate that the patient must not have any living children, any children living in the family home or that patients with children are not excluded, but funding priority would be given to those without children. Marital status may be important but these criteria can also relate to the existence of a stable relationship, sometimes of a certain duration. If no criteria are listed, this indicates that there are no fixed criteria. Waiting times are approximate, and where a range of time was provided the maximum time is shown. Waiting times are not shown where they are unknown due to re-opening of the waiting list, variable according to the treatment required or the clinic carrying out the treatment, or this information was not provided to us by the HA/PCT.

	Airedale PCT	Avon HA	Ayrshire & Arran Health Board	Barking and Havering HA	Barnsley HA	Bedfordshire HA	Berkshire HA	Bexley PCT	Bexley, Bromley & Greenwich HA	Borders Health Board	Bradford City PCT	Bradford South & West PCT	Bromley PCT	Bury & Rochdale HA
TREATMENTS AVAILABLE														
IVF	•	•	•	•	•	•	•	•	•	•			•	•
ICSI	•		•	•	•		•	•	•	•				•
GIFT	•			•	•		•	•	•	•				
IUI	•	•	•	•	•	•	•	•	•	•				
DI	•	•	•	•	•	•	•			•				
tubal surgery	•	•	•	•	•	•	•				•	•		
ovulation induction	•	•	•	•	•	•	•			•	•	•		
embryo freezing	•	•	•		•	•	•						•	
frozen embryo replacement	•	•	•		•	•	•							
other treatment					•									
FUNDING CRITERIA														
married/unmarried		•				•		•					•	•
single women		•	•											
children with partner	•	•	•	•	•	•			•	•	•	•	•	•
including adopted		•	•	•	•					•			•	
children with previous partner	•	•	•	•	•				•	•	•	•	•	•
including adopted		•	•	•	•					•			•	
previous paid treatment						•		•					•	
number of previous treatment cycles		•	•	•	•	•		•	•	•			•	•
length of residence in NHS area														
specific cause of infertility						•							•	
other criteria					•	•				•			•	•
F age max	40	40	39	35	35	35		35	35	38	40	40	38	38
F age min				27	25			28	28					
M age max					55				35				38	
wait in months	-	-	24	15	12	3	-	12	24	0	-	-	-	-

Calderdale & Kirklees HA#	Cambridgeshire HA	Carlisle & District PCT	Central Manchester PCT	County Durham & Darlington HA	Coventry HA	Croydon HA*	Dartford, Gravesham & Swanley PCT	Doncaster HA	Ealing, Hammersmith & Hounslow HA	East Kent HA	East Lancashire HA	East Riding & Hull HA	East Surrey PCT	East Sussex, Brighton and Hove HA#	East Yorkshire PCT	Eastern Health & Soc. Services Board~	Eastern Hull PCT	Forth Valley Health Board	Gateshead & South Tyneside HA
•		•	•	•	•		•	•	•	•	•	•	•	•	•	•	•	•	•
•		•	•	•	•		•	•	•	•	•	•		•	•	•	•	•	•
		•	•	•			•		•		•								
		•	•	•	•			•	•	•	•		•	•		•		•	•
•	•	•	•	•	•			•	•	•	•	•			•	•	•	•	
•			•	•	•			•	•	•				•		•			
•		•	•	•	•	•		•	•	•	•	•		•	•	•	•	•	•
		•	•					•	•	•						•		•	
•		•	•				•	•	•	•	•			•		•		•	
		•				•	•	•	•	•									
		•		•			•				•	•			•		•	•	
		•												•					
•		•	•	•	•		•	•	•	•	•	•	•	•	•	•	•	•	•
•		•		•			•	•			•	•		•	•	•	•	•	•
•		•	•		•		•	•	•	•	•	•	•	•	•	•	•		•
•		•		•			•	•			•			•	•	•	•	•	•
•				•	•								•					•	
•		•		•	•		•	•	•	•	•		•	•		•		•	•
														•		•		•	
				•				•						•	•		•		•
•			•	•	•		•	•				•		•	•	•			
35		36	32	40	37		35	39	36	35	39	35	38	35	35	38	35	38	38
				26			25					25							
35			51	45			60	54			49	46			46		46		
12	18	36	36	-	1.5	-	0	18	6	1.5	24	12	0	-	12	-	12	12	18

	Greater Glasgow Health Board	Gwent HA	Haringey PCT	Herefordshire PCT	Highland Health Board	Hillingdon PCT	Kensington, Chelsea & Westminster HA	Kingston & Richmond HA	Lambeth, Southwark & Lewisham HA	Lanarkshire Health Board	Leeds HA	Lincolnshire HA*	Merton, Sutton & Wandsworth HA	Morecambe Bay PCT
TREATMENTS AVAILABLE														
IVF	•	•	•	•	•	•	•	•	•	•	•	•	•	•
ICSI	•	•	•	•	•	•	•	•	•	•	•	•	•	•
GIFT				•					•	•			•	•
IUI	•	•	•	•		•	•				•	•	•	•
DI	•	•	•	•	•			•	•	•		•	•	•
tubal surgery		•		•					•	•	•	•		•
ovulation induction	•	•	•					•	•	•	•	•	•	
embryo freezing	•	•		•	•				•	•		•		
frozen embryo replacement	•	•			•			•	•	•		•		
other treatment			•							•		•	•	•
FUNDING CRITERIA														
married/unmarried	•				•			•		•				
single women	•	•	•	•						•			•	
children with partner	•	•	•	•	•		•	•		•	•		•	•
including adopted	•	•	•	•	•			•		•				
children with previous partner	•			•	•			•		•				•
including adopted	•			•	•			•		•				
previous paid treatment	•			•	•			•	•	•			•	•
number of previous treatment cycles	•	•	•	•	•	•	•	•	•	•			•	•
length of residence in NHS area	•													
specific cause of infertility	•	•						•		•			•	
other criteria		•	•		•	•	•	•				•		•
F age max	35	36	37	35	37	37	38	35	35	40	34		38	37
F age min										28			25	
M age max	45			55										
wait in months	-	24	18	-	12	-	-	18	-	2.5	12	-	24	15

Newcastle & North Tyneside HA	NHS Orkney	North Bradford PCT	North Cheshire HA	North Derbyshire HA	North Herts & Stevenage PCT*	North Staffordshire HA	North West Lancashire HA	North Yorkshire HA	Northamptonshire HA	Northern Health & Soc. Services Board~	Northumberland HA	Redbridge & Waltham Forest HA*	Rotherham HA	Rushcliffe PCT	Sandwell HA	Sheffield HA	Shropshire HA	Somerset HA*	South Cheshire HA
•	•		•	•	•		•	•		•	•	•	•	•		•	•		•
•			•	•	•		•	•		•	•	•	•	•		•	•		•
•	•		•	•	•	•	•			•	•		•	•		•	•		•
•	•		•	•		•	•	•		•		•	•	•		•	•		•
		•		•		•	•			•	•		•			•		•	•
•	•	•	•	•		•	•	•	•	•	•	•	•	•		•	•	•	•
•	•		•	•			•	•		•		•	•			•		•	•
•	•		•	•			•	•		•		•	•	•		•			•
	•		•			•			•		•			•					
•								•					•	•		•	•		•
•			•										•	•		•	•		•
•	•	•	•	•	•	•	•	•		•	•		•	•		•	•		•
•			•	•	•	•	•	•		•			•	•		•	•		•
•		•	•	•		•		•		•	•		•	•		•	•		•
•			•	•		•	•	•		•			•	•		•	•		•
	•					•	•	•					•	•	•	•			
•	•		•	•		•	•	•		•	•		•	•	•	•			•
•								•							•	•	•		
•					•	•		•		•			•				•		
			•	•	•		•	•		•	•	•	•		•	•			•
40	40	40	36	36		36	37	35		38	35	37	40	35	37	35	-		40
						25					25					25			
		50				45						55	55		55			55
12	0	-	24	18	-	6	-	18	-	-	3	0	18	-	30	24	0	0	48

	South East Hertfordshire PCT**	South Essex HA	South Humber HA	Southern Derbyshire HA	Southern Health & Soc. Services Board~	St Albans & Harpenden PCT	St Helens & Knowsley HA	Trafford North PCT	Wakefield HA	Welwyn & Hatfield PCT	West Hull PCT	West Sussex HA	Wigan & Bolton HA	Wiltshire HA
TREATMENTS AVAILABLE														
IVF		•	•	•	•		•	•	•		•	•	•	•
ICSI		•	•	•	•		•	•	•		•		•	•
GIFT				•			•	•	•				•	•
IUI		•	•	•			•					•	•	•
DI			•	•	•	•	•	•	•	•	•			•
tubal surgery		•		•			•	•				•	•	•
ovulation induction		•	•	•	•		•	•			•	•	•	•
embryo freezing				•			•	•	•				•	
frozen embryo replacement			•	•	•		•	•	•				•	
other treatment					•		•			•			•	
FUNDING CRITERIA														
married/unmarried			•				•		•		•			
single women								•	•					•
children with partner	•	•	•	•			•	•	•		•	•	•	•
including adopted		•	•	•			•	•	•		•		•	•
children with previous partner	•	•	•	•			•	•	•		•	•	•	•
including adopted		•	•	•			•	•	•		•		•	•
previous paid treatment	•			•										
number of previous treatment cycles	•	•	•	•			•	•	•			•	•	
length of residence in NHS area			•								•			
specific cause of infertility	•			•	•		•					•		
other criteria			•	•			•	•	•		•	•	•	
F age max		38	40	40	38		37	40	40		35	38	40	35
F age min			20											
M age max			47	50			50	55			46			50
wait in months	-	24	-	-	-	-	16	24	36	-	12	-	24	0

Wirral HA	•		•			•			•	•	•	•	•	•	•	•	•	•	•				36	50	18
Worcestershire HA	•				•	•	•													•			35	55	-
Yorkshire Wolds & Coast PCT	•		•	•	•			•							•						•	•	35	46	12

* = funding provided only in exceptional circumstances

** = funding provided only in exceptional circumstances
 AND type of treatment available is dependent on circumstances

~ = interim funding arrangement in place at time of data collection – review due 2002/3

\# = criteria listed relate to IVF and/or ICSI only

How to compare clinics

In the following pages, we give you details of almost every NHS and private fertility clinic licensed by the HFEA. As well as contact details for the clinic, we give you the name of the clinical director, together with the year of their graduation. A list of consultants is also provided.

NHS The clinic accepts patients funded by the NHS. Your GP will be able to refer you to this clinic for fertility treatment (for which you will have to join a waiting list), although you may still have to pay for some of the treatment yourself.

SF The clinic accepts self-funded or private patients. Self-funding, where you pay the same cost as the NHS would in order to fund your treatment, is designed for patients who don't have NHS funding or for whom the wait for NHS treatment is too long. For some IVF units, the wait for self-funding, while less than for NHS, is still six months to two years.

£ Payment plans are available for self-funded patients, such as interest-free credit cards or payment by instalment (see p.165 for details).

£R This indicates that refunds are offered to self-funded or private patients if a treatment cycle cannot be completed for medical reasons, for example, if too few eggs develop.

🚐 A satellite or transport IVF service is available. This means that if you live a long way from the clinic at which you will have your embryo transfer, you will be able to have fertility drug treatment at a clinic nearer your home. Egg collection may take place at the satellite clinic or the IVF clinic. However, embryo transfer will always take place at the IVF clinic.

Any drugs required during treatment *do not* have to be purchased at the clinic (although many clinics may provide drugs at reduced cost).

Appears *only* if the clinic can be contacted 24 hours a day in an emergency, for other clinical concerns *and* for advice and emotional support.

Treatments and services

For each clinic, we tell you what treatments and services they provide. There are some abbreviations in the list, as follows:

SO/IUI – superovulation and intra-uterine insemination

DI – donor insemination

IVF w/donor – IVF with donor eggs or sperm

GIFT w/donor – GIFT with donor eggs or sperm

Eligibility criteria

This indicates whether you are likely to be eligible for treatment at the clinic. The 1990 HFEA Act 'does not exclude any woman from being considered for treatment. People seeking treatment are entitled to a fair and unprejudiced assessment of their situation and needs. Treatment may be refused on clinical grounds, or if the fertility clinic believes that it would not be in the interests of any resulting child, or any existing child, to provide treatment.' The eligibility criteria shown are therefore only intended to provide a general indication of the types of patient treated previously at a particular clinic. Patients will be assessed on an individual basis and the decision to treat will take into account many clinical factors, as well as the welfare of the child. NHS patients have to fulfil criteria for funding set by their local PCT.

Guideline age limits for women (F) and men (M) are shown, as are age ranges where these apply. BMI relates to the body mass index of female patients and can be calculated by multiplying your height in metres by itself and dividing your weight in kilograms by the result. For example, if you are 1.6 metres tall and weigh 60kg, the square of your height in metres (1.6x1.6) is 2.56. To get your BMI, divide 60 by 2.56, which gives 23.44.

Costs

Clinics were asked to provide prices for one cycle of IVF and one cycle of IUI with donor sperm, and to indicate if ALL of the following elements of treatment were included in the price provided:

IVF: consultations, scans, blood tests, screening tests, counselling, egg collection, embryo transfer, HFEA fee and drugs.
IUI with donor: consultations, scans, blood tests, screening tests, counselling, HFEA fee and drugs.

Where any element (or part of) is not included, this is listed after the price. For example, 'ONE CYCLE OF IVF £2000 – Not included some/all: consultations, drugs' – indicates that some or all of the consultations and drugs required during treatment are not included in this price, and will therefore incur additional costs. Any additional elements of treatment which *are* included in the price are also shown (where these have been supplied by the clinic). All costs shown are approximate.

Waiting times

Waiting times shown are approximate and patients are advised to contact the clinic directly for confirmation. Times provided in months have been converted to weeks on the basis of one month=four weeks. Where a range of waiting times were provided by the clinic, the maximum time is shown. Where waiting time is not applicable, for example, for NHS patients in a clinic treating only private patients, 'n/a' appears. Where information was not available or provided by the clinic, '-' appears.

Diagnostic tests accepted

Clinics were asked if the results of semen analysis, biochemistry, HIV screening or other diagnostic tests performed outside of the clinic are accepted. Repeat tests may incur additional charges for self-funded or private patients, and may delay the start of treatment.

Support services

Counselling is considered to be so important that every licensed fertility treatment centre in the UK has to provide it by law. Equally, you will need as much support as possible through fertility treatment. We tell you what support services the clinic provides.

These can include independent counselling, independent patient support groups and other support services as specified by the clinic. Some couples prefer to see counsellors that are independent of their treatment. If, for example, the clinic provides counselling by a member of staff such as a fertility nurse, you may feel unable to talk freely about all aspects of your treatment.

Staffing

We tell you what staffing is provided by the clinic. It is preferable to see one physician throughout treatment, have access to a named nurse and a dedicated counsellor (a counsellor who is not otherwise involved in a patient's treatment).

Clinic profile

We asked the clinic to provide any additional information that they felt would be of interest to patients. These profiles also include information about the location of satellite or transport IVF services (where applicable), the nature of any liaison with local GPs and any specific HFEA research licences held.

Methodology

Establishing scope of research and data collection:

Questionnaires were sent to every clinic in the UK licensed by the HFEA. These were developed following focus group research across the country where patients expressed their concerns and talked about the types of information they would like to have access to. The questionnaire was then circulated to leading institutions and organisations, including the Department of Health, CHILD, ISSUE, the Donor Conception Network and ACeBabes. Information regarding the availability of NHS funding, treatments funded and patient eligibility criteria was requested from Health Authorities and PCTs.

Please note that data was not available from the following hospitals and clinics: The Rosie Hospital (Cambridge), Derby City General Hospital, Leicester Royal Infirmary, Dr Louis Hughes (London), St Mary's Hospital (London), St Mary's Hospital (Manchester), Bioscience Centre (Newcastle upon Tyne), Newham General Hospital, Queens Medical Centre (Nottingham), Sheffield Fertility Centre, Royal Infirmary of Edinburgh, Glasgow Nuffield Hospital, Monklands Hospital (Lanarkshire) and Belfast Royal Maternity Hospital.

Assisted Reproduction & Gynaecology Centre

13 Upper Wimpole Street
London
W1G 6LP

PHONE: 020 7486 1230
Clinical Director: Mr Taranissi

(NHS) (SF) (image)

TREATMENTS AND SERVICES
IVF, ICSI, DI, IVF w/donor, egg donation, sperm recovery, assisted
hatching, embryo store, sperm store, egg store

ELIGIBILITY CRITERIA
subject to individual assessment

ONE CYCLE OF IVF £2100
Not included some/all: initial consultation, blood tests, screening tests,
counselling, HFEA fee, drugs

ONE CYCLE OF IUI W/DONOR £475
Not included some/all: initial consultation, blood tests, screening tests,
HFEA fee, drugs

WAITING TIMES IN WEEKS	NHS	PRIVATE
For initial consultation	4	4
To start treatment IVF	0	0
To start treatment IUI w/donor sperm	n/a	n/a

DIAGNOSTIC TESTS ACCEPTED
semen analysis, biochemistry, HIV screen

SUPPORT SERVICES
independent counselling

STAFFING
one physician throughout

CONSULTANTS
Mr Gorgy, Mr Taranissi

The clinic has not provided any further information about its services.

Barts & the London NHS Fertility Centre

Department of Gynaecology
St Bartholomew's Hospital
West Smithfield
London EC1A 7BE

PHONE: 020 7601 7176
Clinical Director: Professor J G
Grudzinskas (1969)

(NHS) (SF) (£R) (🚗) (👤) (24)

TREATMENTS AND SERVICES
IVF, ICSI, SO/IUI, DI, IVF w/donor, egg donation, sperm recovery, tubal
surgery, assisted hatching, embryo store, sperm store, storage of ovarian
tissue

ELIGIBILITY CRITERIA
F 44yrs max, BMI <35

ONE CYCLE OF IVF £1400
Not included some/all: drugs

ONE CYCLE OF IUI W/DONOR £450
Not included some/all: drugs

WAITING TIMES IN WEEKS	NHS	PRIVATE
For initial consultation	6	4
To start treatment IVF	0	0
To start treatment IUI w/donor sperm	0	0

DIAGNOSTIC TESTS ACCEPTED
biochemistry, HIV screen

SUPPORT SERVICES
independent counselling, independent support group

STAFFING
one physician throughout, named nurse system, dedicated counsellor

CONSULTANTS
Mr Talha Al-Shawaf (1976), Mr Colin Davis (1989), Professor J G
Grudzinskas (1969), Mr Adrian Lower (1984)

This clinic is a non profit-making organisation staffed by a multi-
disciplinary team. Staff are available to patients before, during and in the
sometimes difficult months following treatment. In spite of expansion,
staff at the clinic feel that they manage to maintain a personal touch.
A satellite/ transport service is available in Norfolk. GPs are updated
through training and open days.

Bath Assisted Conception Clinic

Forbes Fraser Unit
Royal United Hospital
Combe Park
Bath BA1 3NG

PHONE: 01225 825 560
Clinical Director: Mr Nick Sharp

(NHS) (SF) (£) (R&E) (bottle) (24)

TREATMENTS AND SERVICES
IVF, ICSI, SO/IUI, DI, IVF w/donor, egg donation, sperm recovery, assisted hatching, embryo store, sperm store, embryo donation

ELIGIBILITY CRITERIA
F 43yrs max if using own gametes, established relationship, advice given on BMI, prefer non-smokers, donated eggs not usually offered to those with children or after sterilisation, patients also individually assessed

ONE CYCLE OF IVF £2350
Not included some/all: drugs
Included: 1st yr embryo storage, all follow-up consultations during current treatment and prior to subsequent cycles

ONE CYCLE OF IUI W/DONOR £325 (SUBSEQUENT CYCLES £280)
Not included some/all: gonadotrophins if required are extra

WAITING TIMES IN WEEKS	NHS	PRIVATE
For initial consultation	4	4
To start treatment IVF	0	0
To start treatment IUI w/donor sperm	0	0

DIAGNOSTIC TESTS ACCEPTED
biochemistry, HIV screen

SUPPORT SERVICES
independent counselling, telephone helpline

STAFFING
dedicated counsellor, team of 2 doctors/3 nurses/2 embryologists, nurse-co-ordinated DI and egg/embryo donation programme

CONSULTANTS
Mr Nick Sharp, Mr David Walker

BACC opened in 1994 and is jointly managed by the Royal United Hospital NHS Trust – for whom it co-ordinates the NHS reproductive medicine service – and the privately run BMI Bath Clinic. The clinic carries out approximately 250 fresh treatment cycles a year, as well as a frozen embryo transfer programme. Patients consistently comment that they 'never feel like a number'. Its counselling service is free of charge and can be readily accessed by both NHS and self-funding patients. GPs are updated by newsletter and open days.

Billinge Hospital

Upholland Road
Billinge
Wigan
WN5 7ET

PHONE: 01695 626 485
Clinical Director: Mr C S Chandler
(1975)

NHS **SF** (icon) (24)

TREATMENTS AND SERVICES
GIFT, SO/IUI, DI, GIFT w/donor, egg donation, tubal surgery – IVF and
ICSI for NHS patients only, via transport service at St Mary's Hospital in
Manchester

ELIGIBILITY CRITERIA
NHS patients: F 40yrs max, no existing children, no previous NHS-funded
IVF, smokers advised to stop – self-funded patients individually assessed

ONE CYCLE OF IVF £ N/A
Not included some/all: n/a

ONE CYCLE OF IUI W/DONOR £ N/A
Not included some/all: n/a

WAITING TIMES IN WEEKS	NHS	PRIVATE
For initial consultation	12	-
To start treatment IVF	104	-
To start treatment IUI w/donor sperm	104	0

DIAGNOSTIC TESTS ACCEPTED
biochemistry, HIV screen

SUPPORT SERVICES
independent counselling

STAFFING
named nurse system, dedicated counsellor

CONSULTANTS
Mr C S Chandler (1975)

At the infertility clinic at Billinge Hospital, 2 consultants head a team
of 2 nurses. There is also a specialist nurse appointed to assist the
throughput of the waiting list, which has recently been re-opened.
A counselling service is available for pre-treatment support. The hospital
feels it is important that patients are involved in their treatment and
remain in control of their management. Satellite/transport IVF service
operates at St Mary's Hospital in Manchester.

Birmingham Women's Hospital

Assisted Conception Unit
Edgbaston
Birmingham
B15 2TG

PHONE: 0121 627 2700
Clinical Director: Mr Masoud
Afnan (1980)

NHS   **SF**   **£R**   **(A)**

TREATMENTS AND SERVICES
IVF, ICSI, SO/IUI, DI, IVF w/donor, egg donation, egg sharing, sperm recovery, tubal surgery, embryo store, sperm store, ovulation induction, selective salpingography

ELIGIBILITY CRITERIA
F 50yrs max, 1yr relationship min

ONE CYCLE OF IVF £1650
Not included some/all: drugs

ONE CYCLE OF IUI W/DONOR £350
Not included some/all: drugs

WAITING TIMES IN WEEKS	NHS	PRIVATE
For initial consultation	-	2
To start treatment IVF	-	0
To start treatment IUI w/donor sperm	-	0

DIAGNOSTIC TESTS ACCEPTED
biochemistry, HIV screen

SUPPORT SERVICES
independent counselling, independent support group

STAFFING
one physician throughout, named nurse system, dedicated counsellor

CONSULTANTS
Mr Masoud Afnan (1980), Mr Khaldoun Sharif (1985)

The ACU at Birmingham Women's Hospital aims to provide patients with relevant information and a minimum of tests in order to help them choose the best treatment for them. Diagnostic and therapeutic services are offered for all types of female and male infertility. Many assisted conception techniques used in the UK were developed in the unit, including salpingography, transmyometrial embryo transfer and blastocyst culture. The clinic holds educational meetings for GPs.

Bishop Auckland Fertility Centre

Bishop Auckland General Hospital
Cockton Hill Road
Bishop Auckland
DL14 6AD

PHONE: 01388 454 034
Clinical Director: Mr Robert
Oghoetuoama

(NHS) (SF) (£R) (A) (24)

TREATMENTS AND SERVICES
SO/IUI, DI, tubal surgery, sperm store

ELIGIBILITY CRITERIA
F 40yrs max, M 50yrs max, number of children from current relationship
(not including adopted), length of relationship and history of male or
female sterilisation considered

ONE CYCLE OF IVF £ N/A
Not included some/all: n/a

ONE CYCLE OF IUI W/DONOR £ N/A
Not included some/all: n/a

WAITING TIMES IN WEEKS	NHS	PRIVATE
For initial consultation	-	-
To start treatment IVF	-	-
To start treatment IUI w/donor sperm	-	-

DIAGNOSTIC TESTS ACCEPTED
semen analysis, biochemistry, HIV screen

SUPPORT SERVICES
independent counselling, independent support group

STAFFING
one physician throughout, named nurse system, dedicated counsellor

CONSULTANTS
Mr Robert Oghoetuoama

Bishop Auckland Fertility Centre is a small unit offering ovulation
induction, IUI, DI and DI/IUI. The service is currently under review
following a change of consultant. It is hoped that in the future the
centre will offer a satellite/transport IVF service.

BMI Chaucer Hospital

The Brabourne Suite
Nackington Road
Canterbury
Kent CT4 7AR

PHONE: 01227 825 125
Clinical Director: Mr N M Rafla
(1974)

(NHS) (SF) (£) (®R) (♨) (24)

TREATMENTS AND SERVICES
IVF, ICSI, SO/IUI, DI, IVF w/donor, egg donation, egg sharing, sperm
recovery, tubal surgery, assisted hatching, embryo store, sperm store

ELIGIBILITY CRITERIA
F 42yrs max, relationship 1yr minimum

ONE CYCLE OF IVF £1800
Not included some/all: consultations, blood tests, screening tests, drugs

ONE CYCLE OF IUI W/DONOR £550
Not included some/all: consultations, blood tests, screening tests, drugs

WAITING TIMES IN WEEKS	NHS	PRIVATE
For initial consultation	2	2
To start treatment IVF	8	8
To start treatment IUI w/donor sperm	8	8

DIAGNOSTIC TESTS ACCEPTED
biochemistry, HIV screen

SUPPORT SERVICES
independent counselling

STAFFING
one physician throughout, named nurse system, dedicated counsellor

CONSULTANTS
Mr J O Davies (1975), Mr P W Evans (1987), Mr N M Rafla (1974),
Mr L M A Shaw (1978)

The Chaucer Hospital's ACU opened 6 years ago and performs 300 cycles
a year. It currently holds the local NHS contract for South East Kent as
well as treating an equal number of private patients. Couples are
encouraged to visit the unit on a purely informal basis to discuss their
needs and concerns, to meet the team and view the technical facilities.
Success rates are updated monthly and published for the benefit of
patients and prospective patients.

BMI Chelsfield Park Hospital

Bucks Cross Road
Chelsfield
Orpington
Kent BR6 7RG

PHONE: 01689 877 855
Clinical Director: Miss L Hanna
(1976)

(NHS) (SF) (£) (£R) (🚐) (🜊) (24)

TREATMENTS AND SERVICES
IVF, ICSI, GIFT, SO/IUI, DI, IVF w/donor, sperm recovery, tubal surgery, embryo store, sperm store

ELIGIBILITY CRITERIA
subject to individual assessment

ONE CYCLE OF IVF £2075
Not included some/all: screening tests, drugs

ONE CYCLE OF IUI W/DONOR £730
Not included some/all: screening tests, drugs

WAITING TIMES IN WEEKS	NHS	PRIVATE
For initial consultation	0	0
To start treatment IVF	0	0
To start treatment IUI w/donor sperm	0	0

DIAGNOSTIC TESTS ACCEPTED
biochemistry, HIV screen, laparoscopy, hysteroscopy, hormone profile

SUPPORT SERVICES
independent counselling

STAFFING
one physician throughout, named nurse system, dedicated counsellor

CONSULTANTS
Mr M Ahmed, Mr I Dickinson, Mr J Erian, Miss L Hanna, Mr C Steer

Chelsfield Park Hospital's Assisted Conception Unit is well established and offers in-depth consultation for each couple. After this a treatment plan is tailored to their personal circumstances. Satellite IVF service is offered at Farnborough Hospital and a transport IVF service at Queen Mary's Hospital.

BMI Chiltern Hospital

London Road
Great Missenden
Buckinghamshire
HP16 OEN

PHONE: 01494 892 276
Clinical Director: Dr Julian
Norman-Taylor (1982)

SF **£** **(£R)** **(🍼)** **24**

TREATMENTS AND SERVICES
IVF, ICSI, GIFT, SO/IUI, DI, IVF w/donor, GIFT w/donor, egg donation,
egg sharing, sperm recovery, tubal surgery, assisted hatching, embryo
store, sperm store, minimal access surgery

ELIGIBILITY CRITERIA
subject to individual assessment

ONE CYCLE OF IVF £1995
Not included some/all: blood tests, screening tests, drugs

ONE CYCLE OF IUI W/DONOR £615
Not included some/all: blood tests, screening tests, drugs

WAITING TIMES IN WEEKS	NHS	PRIVATE
For initial consultation	n/a	2
To start treatment IVF	n/a	0
To start treatment IUI w/donor sperm	n/a	0

DIAGNOSTIC TESTS ACCEPTED
biochemistry, HIV screen

SUPPORT SERVICES
independent counselling, independent support group

STAFFING
one physician throughout

CONSULTANTS
Dr Julian Norman-Taylor (1982)

Set in the Buckinghamshire countryside, the Fertility Unit at the Chiltern
Hospital aims to take an individualised and holistic approach to
treatment, whilst trying to reduce the stress associated with it. Self-
referrals are welcomed in addition to those from GPs or gynaecologists.
Couples seeking advice or treatment may attend the clinic on an
informal, free of charge basis to discuss the options available to them
with a nurse. The clinic holds educational meetings for local GPs.

BMI Priory Hospital

Fertility Unit
Priory Road
Edgbaston
Birmingham B5 7UG

PHONE: 0121 440 2323
Clinical Director: Mr R Sawers
(1969)

(NHS) (SF) (£) (🧍) (24)

TREATMENTS AND SERVICES
IVF, ICSI, GIFT, SO/IUI, DI, IVF w/donor, GIFT w/donor, egg donation, egg sharing, sperm recovery, tubal surgery, assisted hatching, embryo store, sperm store, ZIFT, sperm banking prior to vasectomy, chemotherapy or radiotherapy

ELIGIBILITY CRITERIA
F 50yrs max

ONE CYCLE OF IVF £2322
Not included some/all: n/a
Included: pregnancy test, pregnancy scans up to 12 weeks

ONE CYCLE OF IUI W/DONOR £450
Not included some/all: blood tests, screening tests *Included:* pregnancy test, pregnancy scans up to 12 weeks, urine hormone assays

WAITING TIMES IN WEEKS	NHS	PRIVATE
For initial consultation	2	2
To start treatment IVF	0	0
To start treatment IUI w/donor sperm	0	0

DIAGNOSTIC TESTS ACCEPTED
semen analysis, biochemistry, HIV screen, chromosome analysis

SUPPORT SERVICES
independent counselling, independent support group

STAFFING
one physician throughout, dedicated counsellor

CONSULTANTS
Mrs Susan Blunt (1976), Mr R Sawers (1969), Mr Kaldoun W S Sharif (1984), Mr John F Watts (1975)

Established in 1989, the Priory Fertility Unit has 5 consultants which helps to keep waiting times low and provides patients with more choice. Treatment is consultant led. In addition the unit has a team of nurses, embryologists and counsellors. Staff explain the processes involved in treatment and support patients as they undergo investigation and treatment. Open evenings are held each month, enabling patients to visit and get to know the staff involved in providing their care. Interest-free payment arrangements are available on request. The unit holds meetings with GPs annually.

BMI Shirley Oaks Hospital

Fertility Treatment Centre
Poppy Lane, Shirley Oaks Village
Croydon
Surrey CR9 8AB

PHONE: 020 8655 5540
Clinical Director: Mr Michael
W Booker

(SF) (£) (®) (🚐) (👤) (24)

TREATMENTS AND SERVICES
IVF, ICSI, SO/IUI, DI, IVF w/donor, tubal surgery, assisted hatching, sperm store, treatment for gynaecological disease causing infertility eg conservative surgery for endometriosis or myomectomy for uterine fibroids

ELIGIBILITY CRITERIA
F 43yrs max, women may be advised to lose weight and both partners encouraged to stop smoking

ONE CYCLE OF IVF £2200
Not included some/all: screening tests, drugs

ONE CYCLE OF IUI W/DONOR £610 (STIMULATED CYCLE – NATURAL CYCLE £335)
Not included some/all: screening tests, drugs
Included: follow-up consultation with consultant, and/or pregnancy scan

WAITING TIMES IN WEEKS	NHS	PRIVATE
For initial consultation	n/a	3
To start treatment IVF	n/a	8
To start treatment IUI w/donor sperm	n/a	8

DIAGNOSTIC TESTS ACCEPTED
semen analysis, biochemistry, HIV screen, ultrasound scans

SUPPORT SERVICES
independent counselling

STAFFING
one physician throughout, named nurse system, dedicated counsellor

CONSULTANTS
Mr Michael W Booker

The Fertility Treatment Centre at Shirley Oaks Hospital was set up in 1996 by Mr Michael Booker. It is staffed by Mr Booker, his clinical assistant, 2 fertility nurse specialists and an infertility counsellor. Couples usually complete a full investigative work-up before proceeding to treatment. In addition to the treatments offered, the centre offers surgical treatment for a wide range of gynaecological conditions that cause fertility problems, including conservative surgery for endometriosis, myomectomy for uterine fibroids and microsurgical reversal of sterilisation. A satellite/transport IVF service is operated in association with The Bridge Centre. Local GPs are sent regular updates about the centre's services.

Bourn Hall Clinic

Bourn Hall
Bourn
Cambridgeshire
CB3 7TR

PHONE: 01954 719 111
Clinical Director: Mr Peter Brinsden
(1966)

(NHS) (SF) (£R) (🚐) (🧪) (24)

TREATMENTS AND SERVICES
IVF, ICSI, SO/IUI, DI, IVF w/donor, egg donation, egg sharing, sperm recovery, assisted hatching, embryo store, sperm store, egg store, management of spinal cord injured men, embryo donation, IVF surrogacy

ELIGIBILITY CRITERIA
F 45yrs max (48yrs if using donor eggs), 2yr relationship min, BMI<30, no single women or couples of same sex (this policy currently under review)

ONE CYCLE OF IVF £2250
Not included some/all: initial consultation, screening tests, HFEA fee, drugs

ONE CYCLE OF IUI W/DONOR £700
Not included some/all: initial consultation, screening tests, HFEA fee, drugs

WAITING TIMES IN WEEKS	NHS	PRIVATE
For initial consultation	3	3
To start treatment IVF	3	3
To start treatment IUI w/donor sperm	3	3

DIAGNOSTIC TESTS ACCEPTED
all recent and documented tests are accepted

SUPPORT SERVICES
independent counselling, independent support group, newsletter, helpline, website: www.bourn-hall-clinic.co.uk

STAFFING
five infertility specialists, 14 infertility nurses, 5 embryologists, 2 independent counsellors

CONSULTANTS
Mr Peter Brinsden (1966)

Bourn Hall Clinic presently carries out between 1000–1500 treatment cycles per year, including 800–900 IVF cycles and 300 frozen embryo transfer and AI cycles, as well as other treatments including egg donation, IVF surrogacy and the infertility treatment of spinal cord injured men. Over 45 members of staff aim to provide individualised treatment in order to maximise the chances of success. The clinic holds open days for patients, and provides lectures and newsletters to GPs. A satellite/transport IVF service runs at Kings Lynn, Great Yarmouth, Ipswich, Cambridge, Kettering, Jersey and Dublin. A research licence is held for oocyte freezing.

Brentwood Fertility Centre

The Essex Nuffield Hospital
Shenfield Road
Brentwood
Essex CM15 8EH

PHONE: 01277 695 680
Clinical Directors:
Mr A R Haloob (1972)
Mr Satha Sathanandan (1973)

SF **(£R)** **(8)**

TREATMENTS AND SERVICES
IVF, ICSI, SO/IUI, DI, IVF w/donor, egg donation, egg sharing, sperm
recovery, tubal surgery, assisted hatching, embryo store, sperm store,
blastocyst culture, Clomid cycles

ELIGIBILITY CRITERIA
subject to individual assessment

ONE CYCLE OF IVF £1800
Not included some/all: consultations, all scans except pregnancy scan,
blood tests, screening tests, drugs

ONE CYCLE OF IUI W/DONOR £500
Not included some/all: consultations, blood tests, screening tests, drugs

WAITING TIMES IN WEEKS	NHS	PRIVATE
For initial consultation	n/a	1
To start treatment IVF	n/a	0
To start treatment IUI w/donor sperm	n/a	0

DIAGNOSTIC TESTS ACCEPTED
biochemistry, HIV screen (HSG, laproscopy and semen analysis would
probably be repeated)

SUPPORT SERVICES
independent counselling, independent support group

STAFFING
one physician throughout, dedicated counsellor

CONSULTANTS
Mr A R Haloob (1972), Mr Satha Sathanandan (1973)

The Brentwood Fertility Centre opened as a satellite centre in 1994 and
has offered full fertility services since June 2001. Its laboratory is
equipped with the latest technology used in embryology, and has a
team of consultants, nurses and embryologists. GPs are kept up to date
at information evenings.

The Bridge Centre

1 St Thomas Street
London
SE1 9RY

PHONE: 020 7403 3363
Medical Director: Professor J G
Grudzinskas (1969)

TREATMENTS AND SERVICES
IVF, ICSI, GIFT, SO/IUI, DI, IVF w/donor, egg donation, egg sharing,
sperm recovery, tubal surgery, assisted hatching, embryo store, sperm
store, PGD, blastocyst, aneuploidy screening

ELIGIBILITY CRITERIA
subject to individual assessment

ONE CYCLE OF IVF £2375
Not included some/all: initial consultations, scans, screening tests, HFEA
fee, drugs *Included:* 5 ultrasound scans, car service on egg-collection day
and 1 follow-up consultation

ONE CYCLE OF IUI W/DONOR £560 (STIMULATED CYCLE – NATURAL CYCLE £525)
Not included some/all: consultations, screening tests, HFEA fee, drugs

WAITING TIMES IN WEEKS	NHS	PRIVATE
For initial consultation	2	2
To start treatment IVF	0	0
To start treatment IUI w/donor sperm	0	0

DIAGNOSTIC TESTS ACCEPTED
UK tests are normally accepted if performed within the last 6 months by
GP/NHS and with normal results. Other results subject to approval

SUPPORT SERVICES
independent counselling

STAFFING
dedicated counsellor, team approach favoured by clinic director but 1
physician throughout treatment is available upon request

CONSULTANTS
Professor J G Grudzinskas (1969), also see below

The Bridge Centre aims to provide the best possible information and
advice to patients, who are closely involved in the treatment decision
process. It is recognised that the objective of treatment is a successful live
birth, but that realistically this is not possible for every patient. Support
and counselling is based on realism, honesty and humanity. A satellite/
transport service is available at Mayday Hospital, Shirley Oaks Hospital,
Queen Mary Roehampton, St Bartholomew's Hospital, BUPA Roding,
Surrey and Sussex, Maidstone Fertility Centre and Princess Alexandra
Hospital. Consultants: Dr R Balet ('77), Professor A Handyside ('75), Mr
N Perks ('82), Dr E Lammarrone ('94), Ms G Robinson ('85), Mr M Savvas
('82), Ms S Smith ('83), Dr A Watralot ('70) and Dr A Zosmer ('83).

Bristol University

Centre for Reproductive Medicine
4 Priory Road
Clifton
Bristol BS8 1TY

PHONE: 0117 902 1100
Clinical Director: Mr Julian Jenkins

(NHS) (SF) (R£) (🚑) (🍼) (24)

TREATMENTS AND SERVICES
IVF, ICSI, SO/IUI, DI, IVF w/donor, egg donation, sperm recovery, assisted hatching, embryo store, sperm store, infertility investigations, advanced seminology

ELIGIBILITY CRITERIA
BMI <35, donor egg recipients 45yrs max

ONE CYCLE OF IVF £2255
Not included some/all: consultations, screening tests, drugs
Included: consultations during treatment and 1 follow-up, pregnancy scan

ONE CYCLE OF IUI W/DONOR £400
Not included some/all: consultations, screening tests, drugs
Included: consultations during treatment and 1 follow-up, pregnancy scan

WAITING TIMES IN WEEKS	NHS	PRIVATE
For initial consultation	4	4
To start treatment IVF	0	0
To start treatment IUI w/donor sperm	0	0

DIAGNOSTIC TESTS ACCEPTED
biochemistry, HIV screen

SUPPORT SERVICES
independent counselling, independent support group,
website: www.reproMed.co.uk

STAFFING
one physician throughout, named nurse system, dedicated counsellor

CONSULTANTS
Dr David Cahill, Dr Uma Deve Gordon, Mr Julian Jenkins

Opened in 1983, the Centre has seen more than 2000 babies born to couples with fertility problems. In addition to clinical services to diagnose and treat infertility, it runs an ongoing research programme which aims to understand its causes. All services are provided under one roof and patients usually see their own nominated specialist nurse and doctor at every stage of treatment. The Centre also provides newsletters, updates and study days for GPs. A satellite/transport IVF service operates at Taunton & Somerset Hospital and Winfield Hospital, Gloucester.

Burton Centre for Reproductive Medicine

Outwoods House
Queen's Hospital, Belvedere Road
Burton upon Trent
Staffordshire DE13 0RB

PHONE: 01283 566 333 ext. 2387
Clinical Director: Mr Kevin Artley
(1984)

TREATMENTS AND SERVICES
IVF, ICSI, SO/IUI, DI, IVF w/donor, egg donation, egg sharing, sperm
recovery, assisted hatching, embryo store, sperm store, egg store,
oocyte freezing

ELIGIBILITY CRITERIA
preferred ages of private patients: F 45ys or less, M 55yrs or less,
NHS patient criteria as per local PCT

ONE CYCLE OF IVF £1500
Not included some/all: drugs

ONE CYCLE OF IUI W/DONOR £450
Not included some/all: drugs

WAITING TIMES IN WEEKS	NHS	PRIVATE
For initial consultation	8	4
To start treatment IVF	156	8
To start treatment IUI w/donor sperm	156	8

DIAGNOSTIC TESTS ACCEPTED
biochemistry, HIV screen, Hep B/C result if from last 6 months

SUPPORT SERVICES
independent counselling, independent support group

STAFFING
one physician throughout, named nurse system, dedicated counsellor

CONSULTANTS
Mr Kevin Artley (1984)

The BCRM is a newly created patient-orientated unit, staffed by a small
consultant-led team. The clinic is located in a self-contained unit off the
main hospital, offering privacy and comfort. It has 'state of the art'
laboratory facilities designed to exceed statutory requirements for health
and safety. The clinic holds regular meetings with GPs, and provides
them with updates on College guidelines and referral criteria.

CARE at the Alexandra Hospital

Victoria Park
108–112 Daisy Bank Road
Manchester
M1 5QH

PHONE: 0161 257 3799
Clinical Director: Mr Glenn
Atkinson (1983)

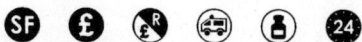

(SF) (£) (®) (🚌) (🛏) (24)

TREATMENTS AND SERVICES
IVF, ICSI, GIFT, SO/IUI, DI, IVF w/donor, GIFT w/donor, egg donation,
egg sharing, sperm recovery, tubal surgery, assisted hatching, embryo
store, sperm store, egg store, blastocyst transfer

ELIGIBILITY CRITERIA
subject to individual assessment

ONE CYCLE OF IVF £1986
Not included some/all: initial consultation (additional £130), screening
tests, drugs

ONE CYCLE OF IUI W/DONOR £470
Not included some/all: consultations, screening tests, drugs

WAITING TIMES IN WEEKS	NHS	PRIVATE
For initial consultation	n/a	4
To start treatment IVF	n/a	0
To start treatment IUI w/donor sperm	n/a	0

DIAGNOSTIC TESTS ACCEPTED
biochemistry, HIV screen, semen tests accepted if performed in specialist
infertility centre

SUPPORT SERVICES
independent counselling, independent support group

STAFFING
one physician throughout, dedicated counsellor

CONSULTANTS
Mr Glenn Atkinson (1983), Mr Rashmikent Patel (1975)

CARE at the Alexandra Hospital aims to offer a comprehensive assisted
conception service from diagnosis to treatment, and ensure that every
aspect of treatment is undertaken by consultants. Members of the team
are pioneers in many treatment advances, including establishing
microinjection technology for male factor infertility. The Alexandra
Hospital is part of the General Healthcare Group and is located near the
centre of Manchester. Sited in a quiet area, treatment is provided in
pleasant and comfortable surroundings. Satellite/transport service is
available at the Beaumont Hospital in Bolton.

CARE at the Park Hospital

Sherwood Lodge Drive
Arnold
Nottingham
NG5 8RX

PHONE: 0115 967 1670
Clinical Director: Mr Simon
Thornton (1979)

(NHS) (SF) (£) (£R) (🚐) (🧴)

TREATMENTS AND SERVICES
IVF, ICSI, SO/IUI, DI, IVF w/donor, egg donation, egg sharing, sperm recovery, tubal surgery, assisted hatching, embryo store, sperm store, egg store, PGD, ovarian tissue freezing

ELIGIBILITY CRITERIA
couples must live at the same address, all are individually assessed and any concerns referred to the clinic's ethics committee

ONE CYCLE OF IVF £1900
Not included some/all: consultations, blood tests, screening tests, drugs
Included: pregnancy test, pregnancy scan and review consultation

ONE CYCLE OF IUI W/DONOR £550
Not included some/all: consultations, screening tests, drugs

WAITING TIMES IN WEEKS	NHS	PRIVATE
For initial consultation	4	4
To start treatment IVF	0	0
To start treatment IUI w/donor sperm	0	0

DIAGNOSTIC TESTS ACCEPTED
semen analysis, biochemistry, HIV screen

SUPPORT SERVICES
independent counselling, independent support group, bulletin board, website: www.care-ivf.com

STAFFING
dedicated counsellor

CONSULTANTS
Mr Kenneth Dowell (1981), Dr Simon Fishel (1975), Mr George Ndukwe (1978), Mr Simon Thornton (1979), Mr John Webster

CARE at the Park Hospital was founded in 1997 and aims to become a centre of excellence in the treatment of infertile patients and research into infertility. Patients are only seen and treated by experienced consultants dedicated solely to fertility management. All tests are carried out in-house and the facilities include a dedicated IVF theatre and embryology laboratory. Satellite IVF services are offered at Leicester Nuffield Hospital, Fitzwilliam Hospital, Peterborough and Derby City Hospital. GPs are kept up-to-date by regular updates, meetings and lectures.

CARE at the Three Shires

The Avenue
Cliftonville
Northampton
NN1 5DR

PHONE: 01604 601 606
Clinical Director: Mr Kamel
Mohamed

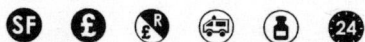

SF **£** **®£** **🚑** **🍼** **24**

TREATMENTS AND SERVICES
IVF, ICSI, GIFT, SO/IUI, DI, IVF w/donor, GIFT w/donor, egg donation, egg sharing, sperm recovery, tubal surgery, assisted hatching, embryo store, sperm store, egg store

ELIGIBILITY CRITERIA
relationship min 1yr, preferable BMI<35, advice given to smokers

ONE CYCLE OF IVF £1750
Not included some/all: consultations, blood tests, screening tests *Included:* down-regulation blood tests, follow-up appointment or pregnancy scan

ONE CYCLE OF IUI W/DONOR £600
Not included some/all: consultations, screening tests, drugs
Included: follow-up appointment or pregnancy scan

WAITING TIMES IN WEEKS	NHS	PRIVATE
For initial consultation	n/a	2
To start treatment IVF	n/a	4
To start treatment IUI w/donor sperm	n/a	4

DIAGNOSTIC TESTS ACCEPTED
HIV screen

SUPPORT SERVICES
independent counselling, independent support group

STAFFING
named nurse system, dedicated counsellor

CONSULTANTS
Mr Roy Davies, Mr Kamel Mohamed

Established in 1989, CARE at the Three Shires is located in purpose-built accommodation within the Three Shires Hospital, itself situated in 100 acres of parkland. The Medical Director has a particular interest in male factor infertility and has held dedicated NHS fertility clinics for many years. Members of the team helped pioneer many treatment advances, including microinjection technology for male factor infertility. All aspects of patient care at the clinic is undertaken by consultants. A satellite/transport service is offered at the Park Hospital, Nottingham.

Centre for Reproductive Medicine, Coventry

University Hospitals Coventry
& Warwickshire NHS Trust
Clifford Bridge Road
Coventry CV2 2DX

PHONE: 024 7653 5167
Clinical Director: Mr Richard
Kennedy (1976)

(NHS) (SF) (£) (£R) (🚑) (🧴) (24)

TREATMENTS AND SERVICES
IVF, ICSI, GIFT, SO/IUI, DI, IVF w/donor, GIFT w/donor, egg donation,
egg sharing, sperm recovery, tubal surgery, assisted hatching, embryo
store, sperm store, egg store, full diagnostic assessments, minimal access
surgery for endometriosis and fibroids etc, blastocyst culture and transfer

ELIGIBILITY CRITERIA
F 49yrs max

ONE CYCLE OF IVF £1495
Not included some/all: drugs *Included:* assisted hatching/blastocyst culture,
embryo freezing/1st years embryo storage, emergency care if required

ONE CYCLE OF IUI W/DONOR £440
Not included some/all: n/a *Included:* additional investigations, admission
and care by the same team for any complications

WAITING TIMES IN WEEKS	NHS	PRIVATE
For initial consultation	10	0
To start treatment IVF	12	0
To start treatment IUI w/donor sperm	-	-

DIAGNOSTIC TESTS ACCEPTED
biochemistry, HIV screen, endocrine, HSG, Hy Cosy, some laparoscopy

SUPPORT SERVICES
independent counselling, independent support group

STAFFING
one physician throughout, genetic nurse counsellor, male reproductive
surgeon, pregnancy counsellor

CONSULTANTS
Mr A R E Blacklock (1969), Mr S Keay (1987), Mr Richard Kennedy
(1976), Mr P Vanekerckhove (1984)

Coventry Centre for Reproductive Medicine was founded by a group of
NHS midwives and patients who felt a full range of treatments should be
available on the NHS. Initial investigations, consultations and tests are
available to all patients on the NHS. Three consultants offer continuity of
care and provide treatments including minimal access surgery. Referrals
from a GP or local consultant are usually required, but direct enquiries are
also welcome. The centre runs training days for practice nurses, lectures for
GPs, study days, an MSc course and postgrad meetings. Satellite/transport
service at Shrewsbury. Research licences are held for in vitro maturation,
oocyte biology, embryo survival after cryopreservation and poor response
to ovarian stimulation. The centre was awarded a Chartermark in 1999.

Centre for Reproductive Medicine & Fertility

The Jessop Wing, Tree Root Walk
Sheffield Teaching Hospitals
NHS Trust
Sheffield S10 2SF

PHONE: 0114 226 8050
Clinical Director: Mr Jonathan Skull
(1988)

TREATMENTS AND SERVICES
IVF, ICSI, GIFT, SO/IUI, DI, IVF w/donor, egg donation, egg sharing,
sperm recovery, tubal surgery, assisted hatching, embryo store, sperm
store, host surrogacy

ELIGIBILITY CRITERIA
subject to individual assessment with particular regard to age and weight

ONE CYCLE OF IVF £1750
Not included some/all: n/a
Included: all pregnancy scans, all drugs required for treatment

ONE CYCLE OF IUI W/DONOR £270 (NATURAL CYCLE – STIMULATED CYCLE £590)
Not included some/all: n/a but additional charges incurred if sperm is
imported from another source

WAITING TIMES IN WEEKS	NHS	PRIVATE
For initial consultation	12	4
To start treatment IVF	104	0
To start treatment IUI w/donor sperm	104	0

DIAGNOSTIC TESTS ACCEPTED
biochemistry, HIV screen, cystic fibrosis screen, HSG, karyotype

SUPPORT SERVICES
independent counselling, independent support group being set up

STAFFING
dedicated counsellor, clinic aims for continuity of care throughout
treatment

CONSULTANTS
Mr Harry Lashen (1982), Professor William L Ledger (1985), Mr T C Li
(1980), Mr Jonathan Skull (1988)

The purpose-built Centre for Reproductive Medicine & Fertility, located
in the new £24 million Jessop Wing, is one of the only fully NHS
managed centres of its kind in the country. Run on a non-profit-making
basis, fees include all treatment-related costs with no registration fees or
hidden charges. Drugs are included in treatment prices and costs are
reduced if they are prescribed by the patient's GP. Care is consultant led
and emphasis is placed on providing an individual pathway of care and
treatment. All investigative procedures are carried out through the NHS
infertility clinic, although private tests can be arranged through clinic
consultants. A research licence is held for embryo development and
implantation, and embryo stem cell research.

Chelsea & Westminster Hospital

Assisted Conception Unit
369 Fulham Road
London
SW10 9NH

PHONE: 020 8746 8585
Clinical Director: Dr Carole Gilling-Smith (1984)

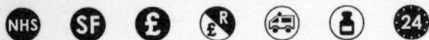

(NHS) (SF) (£) (R£) (🚑) (👤) (24)

TREATMENTS AND SERVICES
IVF, ICSI, SO/IUI, DI, IVF w/donor, egg donation, sperm recovery, assisted hatching, embryo store, sperm store, blastocyst culture and sperm washing for HIV positive men, IVF, ICSI and embryo storage for Hep B/C and HIV affected patients

ELIGIBILITY CRITERIA
F 45yrs max, relationship min 1yr, BMI < 40

ONE CYCLE OF IVF £1880
Not included some/all: drugs
Included: 2 early pregnancy scans if successful

ONE CYCLE OF IUI W/DONOR £400
Not included some/all: consultations, drugs

WAITING TIMES IN WEEKS	NHS	PRIVATE
For initial consultation	6	6
To start treatment IVF	0	0
To start treatment IUI w/donor sperm	0	0

DIAGNOSTIC TESTS ACCEPTED
biochemistry, HIV screen, lap & dye, hysteroscopy, hysterosalpingogram

SUPPORT SERVICES
independent counselling

STAFFING
named nurse system, dedicated counsellor

CONSULTANTS
Mr Hossam Abdulla (1977), Dr Carole Gilling-Smith (1984), Dr Julian Norman-Taylor (1982), Mr Jonathan W Ramsey (1977)

This ACU provides a combined approach to infertility. Both partners are screened for a treatable factor during 2 consultations a month or so apart. Baseline diagnostic tests are arranged prior to initial consultation and this is used to focus on any abnormal test results. A comprehensive treatment plan is formed by a gynaecologist/male infertility specialist team. This is the only fertility centre in the UK with a dedicated laboratory for handling infectious samples and it offers pre-conceptual counselling and treatment for couples where one or both partners are infected with HIV and Hepatitis B/C. Sperm washing techniques have resulted in the birth of 8 healthy children to date. A satellite IVF/ICSI service available for hepatitis B/C and HIV affected patients at the BMI Chiltern Hospital.

Cleveland Gynaecology & Fertility Centre

Spring House
Great Broughton
Stokesley
Cleveland TS9 7HX

PHONE: 01642 778 239
Clinical Director: Mr Philip Taylor

SF **£R** **(I)** **24**

TREATMENTS AND SERVICES
SO/IUI, DI

ELIGIBILITY CRITERIA
F 45yrs max

ONE CYCLE OF IVF £ N/A
Not included some/all: n/a

ONE CYCLE OF IUI W/DONOR £270
Not included some/all: consultations, scans, blood tests, screening tests, counselling, drugs

WAITING TIMES IN WEEKS	NHS	PRIVATE
For initial consultation	n/a	2
To start treatment IVF	n/a	0
To start treatment IUI w/donor sperm	n/a	0

DIAGNOSTIC TESTS ACCEPTED
semen analysis, biochemistry

SUPPORT SERVICES
independent counselling, independent support group

STAFFING
care is delivered by 1 of 2 physicians

CONSULTANTS
Mr Fayez Mustafa, Mr Philip Taylor

This is a small private clinic set in the North Yorkshire moors. It provides a donor insemination service for patients from a wide area in the North of England and Scotland. Subject to welfare assessments required by the HFEA, the clinic will treat single women and lesbian couples. It is closely affiliated with the Department of Reproductive Medicine at the James Cook University Hospital, through which a full range of treatments is available including IVF, ICSI and treatments using donor eggs.

The Cromwell IVF and Fertility Centre

Cromwell Hospital
Cromwell Road
London
SW5 0TU

PHONE: 020 7460 5713
Clinical Director: Mr Eric Simons
(1961)

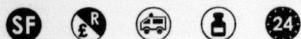

SF **R£** **⊕** **🔋** **24**

TREATMENTS AND SERVICES
IVF, ICSI, GIFT, SO/IUI, DI, IVF w/donor, GIFT w/donor, egg donation, egg sharing, sperm recovery, tubal surgery, assisted hatching, embryo store, sperm store

ELIGIBILITY CRITERIA
F 58yrs max if using donor eggs, weight loss advised if BMI>30, egg donors must have stopped smoking for 3 months

ONE CYCLE OF IVF £2850 (CURRENTLY UNDER REVIEW)
Not included some/all: blood tests, screening tests

ONE CYCLE OF IUI W/DONOR £660
Not included some/all: blood tests, screening tests

WAITING TIMES IN WEEKS	NHS	PRIVATE
For initial consultation	n/a	3
To start treatment IVF	n/a	0
To start treatment IUI w/donor sperm	n/a	0

DIAGNOSTIC TESTS ACCEPTED
biochemistry, HIV screen

SUPPORT SERVICES
independent counselling, independent support group

STAFFING
small team of 3 consultants and 3 nurses – patients are offered consultations with a doctor of their choice

CONSULTANTS
Dr Kamal Ahuja, Miss Ajit Gill (1979), Mr Michael Rimington (1985), Mr Eric Simons (1961)

The Centre pioneered the concept of egg sharing in the UK and successfully persuaded the HFEA to incorporate it into the National Code of Practice. Currently the programme is one of the largest egg sharing services in Europe.

Diana, Princess of Wales Centre for Repro. Medicine

St George's Hospital NHS Trust
3rd Floor, Lanesborough Wing
Cranmer Terrace
London SW17 0RE

PHONE: 020 8725 3308
Clinical Director: Dr Geeta
Nargund (1983)

(NHS) (SF) (£) (£R) (🚐) (🍼) (24)

TREATMENTS AND SERVICES
IVF, ICSI, SO/IUI, DI, IVF w/donor, egg donation, egg sharing, sperm
recovery, assisted hatching, embryo store, sperm store, egg store, natural
cycle IVF, 'one stop' fertility diagnosis

ELIGIBILITY CRITERIA
F 50yrs max, relationship 1yr min

ONE CYCLE OF IVF £1145
Not included some/all: blood tests, screening tests, HFEA fee, drugs
Included: review consultation, pregnancy scans up to 2 weeks

ONE CYCLE OF IUI W/DONOR £495
Not included some/all: blood tests, screening tests, HFEA fee, drugs
Included: donor sperm sample

WAITING TIMES IN WEEKS	NHS	PRIVATE
For initial consultation	4	4
To start treatment IVF	76	0
To start treatment IUI w/donor sperm	76	0

DIAGNOSTIC TESTS ACCEPTED
semen analysis, biochemistry, HIV screen

SUPPORT SERVICES
independent counselling, independent support group, nurse telephone
line, IVF videos/booklets, patient suggestion box

STAFFING
named nurse system, dedicated counsellor, treatment with 1 physician as
far as possible

CONSULTANTS
Dr Geeta Nargund (1983)

Using a patient-centred approach, the Centre offers a 'one stop' fertility
diagnosis service, natural cycle IVF and the use of minimal stimulation for
IVF and ICSI treatments. The clinic regularly runs patient information
evenings on fertility awareness, assisted conception and polycystic ovary
syndrome. The clinical director works as a medical adviser to patient
support groups and is an advocate of cost-effective treatment on the
NHS. Satellite/transport services are offered at Ipswich Hospital and
Create Health Clinic, London.

Elizabeth Garrett Anderson Hospital

Reproductive Medicine Unit
Huntley Street
London
WC1E 6DH

PHONE: 020 7380 9759
Clinical Director: information not
provided by the clinic

NHS ⊕

TREATMENTS AND SERVICES
SO/IUI, DI, tubal surgery, sperm store, ovulation induction, laparoscopic
& hysteroscopic surgery

ELIGIBILITY CRITERIA
clinic offers investigation and counselling – but not treatment – to
women over 40yrs with GP's referral

ONE CYCLE OF IVF £ N/A
Not included some/all: n/a

ONE CYCLE OF IUI W/DONOR £ N/A
Not included some/all: n/a

WAITING TIMES IN WEEKS	NHS	PRIVATE
For initial consultation	16	n/a
To start treatment IVF	0	n/a
To start treatment IUI w/donor sperm	0	n/a

DIAGNOSTIC TESTS ACCEPTED
semen analysis, biochemistry, HIV screen, HSG

SUPPORT SERVICES
independent counselling, hospital provides full gynaecological and
obstetrics service

STAFFING
dedicated counsellor, team approach

CONSULTANTS
Mr E Saridogan (1985)

The Reproductive Medicine Unit provides a comprehensive fertility
service from initial investigation onwards but it does not offer IVF or ICSI.
There are daily consultant clinics, as well as dedicated daily clinics for
patients needing donor insemination and ovulation induction.
Consultants at the unit have special interests including endocrinology,
male subfertility, diagnostic and tubal reconstructive surgery and
ovulation induction. The team includes specialist fertility nurses, full-time
specialist ultrasonographers, laboratory staff, a full-time secretary, clerical
staff, and 2 clinical psychologists providing counselling.

Esperance Private Hospital

Assisted Conception Unit
Hartington Place
Eastbourne
East Sussex BN21 3BG

PHONE: 01323 410 333
Clinical Director: Mr David
Robertson (1977)

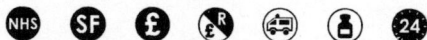

NHS SF £ ®£ 🚐 👤 24

TREATMENTS AND SERVICES
IVF, ICSI, GIFT, SO/IUI, DI, IVF w/donor, GIFT w/donor, egg donation,
sperm recovery, assisted hatching, embryo store, sperm store, IVF
surrogacy, MESA, TESA, ZIFT

ELIGIBILITY CRITERIA
length of relationship considered, female patients must be
pre-menopausal

ONE CYCLE OF IVF £2340
Not included some/all: consultations, drugs
Included: pregnancy scan

ONE CYCLE OF IUI W/DONOR £385
Not included some/all: consultations, blood tests, screening tests, drugs
Included: pregnancy scan

WAITING TIMES IN WEEKS	NHS	PRIVATE
For initial consultation	4	4
To start treatment IVF	0	0
To start treatment IUI w/donor sperm	0	0

DIAGNOSTIC TESTS ACCEPTED
biochemistry, HIV screen

SUPPORT SERVICES
independent counselling, independent support group

STAFFING
one physician throughout, dedicated counsellor

CONSULTANTS
Mr David Robertson (1977)

The Esperance ACU opened in 1989, initially offering artificial insemination treatments with either partner or donor sperm. The first IVF cycle
was carried out in 1990 and the unit is now a modern, fully equipped
facility with close links to local NHS hospitals. The unit recognises that
patients face treatment that is often invasive and stressful. The Director
has specialised in infertility treatment since 1984 and worked for 3 years
with Professor Ian Craft at the Humana Hospital Wellington in London,
then one of the busiest fertility clinics in the world. A satellite/transport
IVF service is available at Haywards Heath, Chichester.

Essex Fertility Centre

Holly House Hospital
High Road
Buckhurst Hill
Essex IG9 5HX

PHONE: 020 8505 3315
Clinical Director: Mr Michael
Ah-Moye (1977)

(SF) (£R) (🚐) (👤) (24)

TREATMENTS AND SERVICES
IVF, ICSI, GIFT, SO/IUI, DI, IVF w/donor, GIFT w/donor, egg donation,
egg sharing, sperm recovery, assisted hatching, embryo store, sperm
store

ELIGIBILITY CRITERIA
F 50yrs max

ONE CYCLE OF IVF £2100
Not included some/all: consultations, blood tests, screening tests, counselling, HFEA fee, drugs *Included:* 1hr session with holistic therapist

ONE CYCLE OF IUI W/DONOR £650
Not included some/all: consultations, blood tests, screening tests, HFEA
fee, drugs *Included:* donor sperm and preparation

WAITING TIMES IN WEEKS	NHS	PRIVATE
For initial consultation	n/a	8
To start treatment IVF	n/a	0
To start treatment IUI w/donor sperm	n/a	0

DIAGNOSTIC TESTS ACCEPTED
semen analysis, biochemistry, HIV screen, hysterosalpinogram,
laparoscopy

SUPPORT SERVICES
independent counselling, independent support group

STAFFING
dedicated counsellor, small team of 2 consultants and 2 nurse
co-ordinators

CONSULTANTS
Mr M Ah-Moye (1977), Mr W Fiamanya (1973), Dr D Viniker (1971)

Founded in 1989, the Essex Fertility Centre was the first fertility clinic
to be established in Essex, Hertfordshire and North East London. Staff
include 2 full-time clinicians with a combined IVF experience of almost
35 years. All egg collections are undertaken in a fully equipped operating
theatre dedicated to IVF, thereby allowing every patient access to general
anaesthetic. Most patients have private room facilities post egg collection
and embryo transfer. Every IVF patient is offered a free 1hr session with a
holistic therapist. The centre runs a regular course of lectures and study
days for GPs. A satellite/transport service is available at the Vivera Clinic,
St John's Wood, London.

Guy's & St Thomas' Hospital

Assisted Conception Unit
4th Floor, Thomas Guy House
Guy's Hospital, St Thomas Street
London SE1 9RT

PHONE: 020 7960 5598
Clinical Director: Dr Alison Taylor

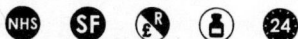

(NHS) (SF) (£R) (👤) (24)

TREATMENTS AND SERVICES
IVF, ICSI, SO/IUI, DI, IVF w/donor, sperm recovery, tubal surgery, assisted
hatching, embryo store, sperm store, PGD

ELIGIBILITY CRITERIA
subject to individual assessment

ONE CYCLE OF IVF £1450
Not included some/all: drugs

ONE CYCLE OF IUI W/DONOR £375
Not included some/all: drugs

WAITING TIMES IN WEEKS	NHS	PRIVATE
For initial consultation	8	8
To start treatment IVF	12	12
To start treatment IUI w/donor sperm	24	24

DIAGNOSTIC TESTS ACCEPTED
biochemistry, HIV screen

SUPPORT SERVICES
independent counselling, independent support group, monthly patient
information evenings

STAFFING
consultant-led service working with a team of nurse practitioners

CONSULTANTS
Professor Peter Braude, Mr Yakoub Khalas, Mr Laurence Mascarenhas,
Dr Alison Taylor

Guy's & St Thomas' Assisted Conception Unit moved into a new
purpose-built unit in Guy's Hospital in 2001. It is staffed by a team of
subspecialty consultants, nurse practitioners, scientific and administrative
staff, providing patients with rapid access to expert advice and as much
support as possible during and after treatment. Regular audit meetings
are held in an effort to continually review practice and improve services.
A research licence is held for pre-implantation genetic diagnosis and
stem cell research.

The Harley Street Fertility Centre

122 Harley Street
London
W1G 7JP

PHONE: 020 7935 2234
Clinical Director: Mr R K Goswamy
(1976)

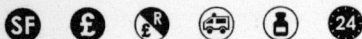

SF **£** **®** **🚗** **💊** **24**

TREATMENTS AND SERVICES
IVF, ICSI, GIFT, SO/IUI, DI, IVF w/donor, GIFT w/donor, egg donation, egg sharing, sperm recovery, tubal surgery, assisted hatching, embryo store, sperm store, doppler studies, 3D ultrasound, investigations for failed IVF and 'unexplained infertility'

ELIGIBILITY CRITERIA
F 44yrs max

ONE CYCLE OF IVF £2400
Not included some/all: consultations, screening tests, drugs

ONE CYCLE OF IUI W/DONOR £500
Not included some/all: consultations, screening tests, drugs

WAITING TIMES IN WEEKS	NHS	PRIVATE
For initial consultation	n/a	1
To start treatment IVF	n/a	0
To start treatment IUI w/donor sperm	n/a	0

DIAGNOSTIC TESTS ACCEPTED
semen analysis, biochemistry, HIV screen

SUPPORT SERVICES
independent counselling, independent support group

STAFFING
one physician throughout, dedicated counsellor

CONSULTANTS
Mr R K Goswamy (1976), Mr M D Kini (1964)

Staff at the Harley Street Fertility Centre have more than 70 years combined experience in IVF and related treatments. They specialise in the investigation of unexplained infertility and failed IVF, and 70 per cent of their patients are in these categories at time of referral. Satellite/transport IVF services is available at BUPA Dunedin Hospital, Reading.

Hartlepool General Hospital

The Cameron Unit
Holdforth Road
Hartlepool
TS24 9SH

PHONE: 01429 522 866
Clinical Director: Mr M
Menabawey (1968)

(NHS) (SF) (R) (b)

TREATMENTS AND SERVICES
IVF, GIFT, SO/IUI, DI, IVF w/donor, tubal surgery, embryo store

ELIGIBILITY CRITERIA
F 39yrs (NHS) max (50yrs for private patients if FSH level is less than
15 u/L), M 55yrs max, NHS patients must have no existing children,
minimum 3yr relationship, maximum 1 previous treatment cycle

ONE CYCLE OF IVF £2300
Not included some/all: drugs

ONE CYCLE OF IUI W/DONOR £270
Not included some/all: drugs

WAITING TIMES IN WEEKS	NHS	PRIVATE
For initial consultation	10	2
To start treatment IVF	26	6
To start treatment IUI w/donor sperm	8	4

DIAGNOSTIC TESTS ACCEPTED
semen analysis, biochemistry, HIV screen

SUPPORT SERVICES
independent counselling, independent support group

STAFFING
one physician throughout, named nurse system, dedicated counsellor

CONSULTANTS
Mr M Menabawey (1968)

Hartlepool Hospital Fertility Unit moved to the Cameron Unit in 1991.
With the support of the staff, hospital management and the clinic's
patient action group, the Cameron Unit provides a full range of fertility
services to both local patients and to those in other Health Authorities in
the region. It offers treatment to single women and self-funded patients
are also accepted.

Homerton University Hospital

Fertility Unit
Homerton Row
Hackney
London E9 6SR

PHONE: 020 8510 7660/7638
Clinical Director: Mr Richard
Howell (1976)

(NHS) (SF) (£R) (🍼) (24)

TREATMENTS AND SERVICES
IVF, ICSI, SO/IUI, DI, IVF w/donor, egg donation, sperm recovery, assisted
hatching, embryo store, sperm store

ELIGIBILITY CRITERIA
F 42yrs max, prefer min 2yr relationship, BMI < 32, smokers strongly
encouraged to stop

ONE CYCLE OF IVF £1230
Not included some/all: drugs (drug costs vary between £800 and £1400
dependent on individual dose required)

ONE CYCLE OF IUI W/DONOR £350
Not included some/all: drugs (drug costs vary between £20 and £120
dependent on individual dose required) *Included:* donor sperm sample

WAITING TIMES IN WEEKS	NHS	PRIVATE
For initial consultation	4	4
To start treatment IVF	40	0
To start treatment IUI w/donor sperm	0	0

DIAGNOSTIC TESTS ACCEPTED
biochemistry, HIV screen

SUPPORT SERVICES
independent counselling, website:
www.the-homerton.demon.co.uk/fertility

STAFFING
named nurse system, dedicated counsellor, small team of 2 doctors

CONSULTANTS
Mr Richard Howell (1976)

Homerton University Hospital is a large teaching hospital and the Fertility
Unit is situated within purpose-built premises within hospital grounds.
The Unit is run on a not-for-profit basis and accepts referrals from all over
the country. Patients usually see the same 2 doctors or nurses each visit,
who aim to tailor treatment to the patient's individual needs. The Unit
offers treatment to single women or women in same-sex relationships.
Telephone queries are welcomed and individual visits from prospective
patients are encouraged.

Hull IVF Unit

The Princess Royal Hospital
Saltshouse Road
Hull
HU8 9HE

PHONE: 01482 676 541
Clinical Director: Mr Steve
Maguiness (1981)

NHS SF (£R) 24

TREATMENTS AND SERVICES
IVF, ICSI, GIFT, SO/IUI, DI, IVF w/donor, GIFT w/donor, egg donation,
egg sharing, sperm recovery, tubal surgery, embryo store, sperm store

ELIGIBILITY CRITERIA
subject to individual assessment

ONE CYCLE OF IVF £1600
Not included some/all: initial consultation (£150 extra), drugs
Included: general anaesthetic if required

ONE CYCLE OF IUI W/DONOR £525
Not included some/all: initial consultation (£150 extra), drugs

WAITING TIMES IN WEEKS	NHS	PRIVATE
For initial consultation	13	4
To start treatment IVF	52	0
To start treatment IUI w/donor sperm	52	0

DIAGNOSTIC TESTS ACCEPTED
semen analysis, biochemistry, HIV screen, echovist tubal pathway testing

SUPPORT SERVICES
independent counselling, independent support group

STAFFING
named nurse system, dedicated counsellor

CONSULTANTS
Professor Stephen Killick (1976), Mr Steve Maguiness (1981)

The Unit was established in 1986 as a collaboration between the NHS
and the University of Hull, funded by an NHS research grant. After two
years this expired and the clinic continued on a private basis, funded by
the Hull IVF Trust. In 1996 it began to treat NHS patients. It continues to
work closely with the Departments of Biological Sciences & Medicine and
is active in subfertility research. There are plans to move to the local hospital Trust's new development in 2003. Patients are cared for by a small
team of experienced nursing staff and radiographers. Two consultants
and a research fellow provide medical input and a consultant urologist
and physician are available if required. Patients can obtain support from
staff at all times and there is an independent counselling service.

The Isis Fertility Centre

The Oaks Hospital
Mile End Road
Colchester
Essex CO4 5XR

PHONE: 01206 752 121
Clinical Director: Mr Adrian Lower
(1983)

SF **(£)** **(⊞)** **(24)**

TREATMENTS AND SERVICES
IVF, ICSI, SO/IUI, DI, IVF w/donor, egg donation, egg sharing, sperm
recovery, tubal surgery, assisted hatching, embryo store, sperm store,
egg store, minimal access surgery including laparoscopy and sterilisation
reversal, laser treatment for endometriosis, hysteroscopy

ELIGIBILITY CRITERIA
subject to individual assessment

ONE CYCLE OF IVF £2395
Not included some/all: screening tests, HFEA fee, drugs
Included: embryo freezing

ONE CYCLE OF IUI W/DONOR £588
Not included some/all: blood tests, screening tests, HFEA fee, drugs

WAITING TIMES IN WEEKS	NHS	PRIVATE
For initial consultation	n/a	0
To start treatment IVF	n/a	0
To start treatment IUI w/donor sperm	n/a	0

DIAGNOSTIC TESTS ACCEPTED
biochemistry, HIV screen

SUPPORT SERVICES
independent counselling

STAFFING
one physician throughout, named nurse system, dedicated counsellor

CONSULTANTS
Mr Adrian Lower (1983), Dr C Marfleet (1974), Mr T Omara Boto (1980)

The Isis Fertility Centre is based at the Oaks Hospital, which houses
state-of-the-art operating theatres and the latest imaging and diagnostic
equipment. The Centre's team aim to investigate the causes of infertility
in the shortest possible time, usually in the space of 1 menstrual cycle.
Treatment plans are based on medical history, results of investigations
and take into account social, cultural and financial circumstances.
The centre holds information meetings for GPs and a satellite/transport
service based in London is available.

James Cook University Hospital

Department of
Reproductive Medicine
Marton Road, Middlesborough
Cleveland TS4 3BW

PHONE: 01642 854 856
Clinical Director: Mr Phillip Taylor
(1970)

NHS SF (£R) (👤) (24)

TREATMENTS AND SERVICES
IVF, ICSI, SO/IUI, DI, IVF w/donor, egg donation, egg sharing, sperm
recovery, tubal surgery, assisted hatching, embryo store, sperm store

ELIGIBILITY CRITERIA
F 48yrs max

ONE CYCLE OF IVF £1595
Not included some/all: consultations, blood tests, drugs

ONE CYCLE OF IUI W/DONOR £270
Not included some/all: consultations, scans, blood tests, screening tests,
drugs

WAITING TIMES IN WEEKS	NHS	PRIVATE
For initial consultation	20	2
To start treatment IVF	105	4
To start treatment IUI w/donor sperm	105	4

DIAGNOSTIC TESTS ACCEPTED
biochemistry, HIV screen

SUPPORT SERVICES
independent counselling, independent support group

STAFFING
team approach – 2 physicians, 3 nurses and 2 embryologists

CONSULTANTS
Mr Fayez Mustafa (1983), Mr Phillip Taylor (1970)

The clinic takes both NHS and private patients, and there is a full range
of diagnostic, surgical and assisted conception procedures available. This
includes tubal microsurgery, IVF, ICSI, donor sperm and donor eggs.

James Paget Hospital

Subfertility Unit, Department of
Obstetrics & Gynaecology
Lowestoft Road, Gorleston
Norfolk NR31 6LA

PHONE: 01493 452 366
Clinical Director: Mr P A
Greenwood (1980)

(NHS) (SF) (£R) (🚐) (👤)

TREATMENTS AND SERVICES
SO/IUI, DI, tubal surgery, sperm store, transport IVF/ICSI with embryo
replacement at Bourn Hall Clinic

ELIGIBILITY CRITERIA
F 40yrs max, M 55yrs max, relationship 1yr min, BMI<30, smoking very
strongly discouraged

ONE CYCLE OF IVF £1500
Not included some/all: screening tests, drugs

ONE CYCLE OF IUI W/DONOR £400
Not included some/all: consultations, blood tests, screening tests, drugs

WAITING TIMES IN WEEKS	NHS	PRIVATE
For initial consultation	12	4
To start treatment IVF	40	10
To start treatment IUI w/donor sperm	n/a	10

DIAGNOSTIC TESTS ACCEPTED
semen analysis, biochemistry

SUPPORT SERVICES
independent counselling

STAFFING
one physician throughout, named nurse system, dedicated counsellor

CONSULTANTS
Mr P A Greenwood (1980)

The Subfertility Unit at James Paget Healthcare NHS Trust serves the local
catchment area. Based in a local district hospital, this small unit has good
links with local GPs. It carries out egg retrieval for a transport IVF service,
with embryo replacement at Bourn Hall Clinic.

King's College Hospital

Assisted Conception Unit
7th Floor, Ruskin Wing
Denmark Hill
London SE5 9RS

PHONE: 020 7346 3143
Clinical Director: Mr John Parsons
(1970)

NHS **SF** **R** **(car)** **(bottle)** **24**

TREATMENTS AND SERVICES
IVF, ICSI, SO/IUI, DI, IVF w/donor, egg donation, sperm recovery, tubal
surgery, assisted hatching, embryo store, sperm store, IVF surrogacy

ELIGIBILITY CRITERIA
minimim 1yr relationship, BMI <35, menstrual FSH less then 15 units/litre

ONE CYCLE OF IVF £1375
Not included some/all: initial consultation, blood tests, screening tests,
drugs, additional charge of £150 in 1st cycle for 1st consultation, semen
analysis, menstrual gonadotrophin measurement and transvaginal scan

ONE CYCLE OF IUI W/DONOR £250
Not included some/all: consultations, screening tests, drugs

WAITING TIMES IN WEEKS	NHS	PRIVATE
For initial consultation	-	8
To start treatment IVF	-	16
To start treatment IUI w/donor sperm	-	-

DIAGNOSTIC TESTS ACCEPTED
information not provided

SUPPORT SERVICES
independent counselling, patient liaison co-ordinator, 'buddy' scheme

STAFFING
dedicated counsellor, 1 physician sees patients at outpatient consultations
and during treatment – provided by small team of doctors and nurses – if
problems develop

CONSULTANTS
Dr Ruth Curson (1972), Mr John Parsons (1970), Dr Emma Sowerby (1996)

The ACU at King's College Hospital was established in 1983 and was
the first centre in the UK to provide IVF as an outpatient procedure. It has
a small friendly team of doctors, nurses and embryologists currently
performing around 650 cycles of IVF/ICSI per year. Treatment is managed
in such a way as to minimise the number of visits to the unit during a
cycle. All procedures are performed in the unit and to maximise continuity of care, most day-to-day clinical procedures are performed by a small
team of specially trained nurses. A transport IVF service is available at St
Helier Hospital.

Leeds General Infirmary

Assisted Conception Unit
Clarendon Wing
Belmont Grove
Leeds LS2 9NS

PHONE: 0113 392 6908
Clinical Director: Mr Anthony
Rutherford (1980)

(NHS) (SF) (£) (£R) (🚗) (🧪) (24)

TREATMENTS AND SERVICES
IVF, ICSI, GIFT, SO/IUI, DI, IVF w/donor, GIFT w/donor, egg donation, sperm recovery, tubal surgery, assisted hatching, embryo store, sperm store, egg store, ovulation induction, surrogacy, PGD

ELIGIBILITY CRITERIA
subject to individual assessment

ONE CYCLE OF IVF £1790
Not included some/all: consultations

ONE CYCLE OF IUI W/DONOR £320
Not included some/all: consultations, drugs

WAITING TIMES IN WEEKS	NHS	PRIVATE
For initial consultation	6	4
To start treatment IVF	4	4
To start treatment IUI w/donor sperm	6	6

DIAGNOSTIC TESTS ACCEPTED
biochemistry, HIV screen

SUPPORT SERVICES
independent counselling, independent support group

STAFFING
team nursing approach

CONSULTANTS
Dr Adam Balen (1984), Mr Anthony Rutherford (1980)

The Clarendon Wing unit was established in 1991, and is housed within a large teaching hospital. This provides the opportunity to hold joint clinics with experts in closely aligned specialties, such as urology for complex male problems, genetics for pre-implantation genetic diagnosis, and oncologists looking to preserve fertility in patients with cancer. The RMU supports research and allows developments in the laboratory to be introduced into clinical practice with the minimum of delay. Satellite/transport IVF services are available at Halifax, Bradford, Barrow-in-Furness, Airedale and Isle of Man. The unit runs postgraduate seminars for GPs and holds a research licence for pre-implantation genetic diagnosis and in vitro maturation of immature oocytes.

The Lister Hospital

Assisted Conception Unit
Chelsea Bridge Road
London
SW1W 8RH

PHONE: 020 7730 3417
Clinical Director: Mr Hossam
Abdalla

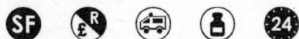

SF **£R** 🚐 🍼 **24**

TREATMENTS AND SERVICES
IVF, ICSI, GIFT, SO/IUI, DI, IVF w/donor, GIFT w/donor, egg donation,
egg sharing, sperm recovery, tubal surgery, assisted hatching, embryo
store, sperm store, egg store

ELIGIBILITY CRITERIA
subject to individual assessment

ONE CYCLE OF IVF £2400
Not included some/all: consultations, blood tests, screening tests, embryo
freezing, HFEA fee, drugs

ONE CYCLE OF IUI W/DONOR £630
Not included some/all: consultations, blood tests, screening tests, HFEA
fee, drugs

WAITING TIMES IN WEEKS	NHS	PRIVATE
For initial consultation	n/a	4
To start treatment IVF	n/a	4
To start treatment IUI w/donor sperm	n/a	4

DIAGNOSTIC TESTS ACCEPTED
biochemistry, HIV screen, hormone analysis

SUPPORT SERVICES
independent counselling, independent support group

STAFFING
one physician throughout, named nurse system, dedicated counsellor

CONSULTANTS
Mr Hossam Abdalla

Established in 1988, the Assisted Conception Unit at The Lister Hospital
carries out over 1400 cycles of IVF and over 200 cycles of ovum donation
every year. The centre has particularly flexible referral criteria in order to
help couples with more difficult fertility problems. Couples are provided
with information and encouraged to be involved in their own treatment.
There are 35 members of clinical and clerical staff. A satellite IVF service
operates at the Sussex Nuffield Hospital in Brighton. Liaison with local
doctors takes place at GP evenings.

Liverpool Women's Hospital

Reproductive Medicine Unit
Crown Street
Liverpool
L8 7SS

PHONE: 0151 702 4123
Clinical Director: Mr Charles
Kingsland (1982)

(NHS) (SF) (R) (🚐) (👤)

TREATMENTS AND SERVICES
IVF, ICSI, SO/IUI, DI, IVF w/donor, egg donation, sperm recovery, assisted
hatching, embryo store, sperm store, egg store

ELIGIBILITY CRITERIA
F 35yrs max (NHS), F 45yrs max (private), no existing children for NHS
patients, min 2yr relationship, BMI<30

ONE CYCLE OF IVF £2600
Not included some/all: n/a

ONE CYCLE OF IUI W/DONOR £500
Not included some/all: n/a

WAITING TIMES IN WEEKS	NHS	PRIVATE
For initial consultation	104	8
To start treatment IVF *after initial consultation*	0	8
To start treatment IUI w/donor sperm	12	12

DIAGNOSTIC TESTS ACCEPTED
biochemistry, HIV screen, tubal function, sperm migration test

SUPPORT SERVICES
independent counselling, independent support group, reflexology, self-
hypnosis, reiki

STAFFING
named nurse system, dedicated counsellor

CONSULTANTS
Mr Charles Kingsland (1982), Dr Lewis-Jones (1972)

The Liverpool Women's Hospital is the largest provider of NHS funded
IVF treatments in the country. The unit provides over 700 NHS and 400
privately funded treatment cycles annually. The Reproductive Medicine
Unit is situated within the Liverpool Women's Hospital, providing full
gynaecological and obstetric back-up facilities for the management of
women and their babies. A full follow-up service is provided for patients
undergoing infertility treatments within the hospital. The clinic offers a
satellite/transport IVF service at Chester, Whiston and Arrowe Park
Hospitals. Local GPs are kept informed by yearly updates. A research
licence is held for andrology factors affecting implantation.

London Female & Male Fertility Centre

Highgate Private Hospital
17–19 View Road
London
N6 4DJ

PHONE: 020 8347 5081
Clinical Director: Mr A Abdel Gadir
(1972)

SF £ (R) (car) (person)

TREATMENTS AND SERVICES
IVF, ICSI, GIFT, SO/IUI, DI, IVF w/donor, GIFT w/donor, egg donation,
sperm recovery, tubal surgery, assisted hatching, embryo store, sperm
store

ELIGIBILITY CRITERIA
F 50yrs max, min 6 months relationship, number of previous cycles and
female weight may be considered in consultation

ONE CYCLE OF IVF £1840
Not included some/all: initial consultation, initial scan, screening tests,
counselling, drugs *Included:* review consultation after treatment

ONE CYCLE OF IUI W/DONOR £675
Not included some/all: initial consultation, initial scan, blood tests, screening tests, counselling, drugs *Included:* review consultation after treatment

WAITING TIMES IN WEEKS	NHS	PRIVATE
For initial consultation	n/a	2
To start treatment IVF	n/a	0
To start treatment IUI w/donor sperm	n/a	0

DIAGNOSTIC TESTS ACCEPTED
biochemistry, HIV screen, Hep B/C, chlamydia

SUPPORT SERVICES
independent counselling, translator available for certain languages by
prior arrangement

STAFFING
one physician throughout, named nurse system, dedicated counsellor

CONSULTANTS
Mr A Abdel Gadir (1972)

The London Female & Male Fertility Centre at Highgate Private Hospital
offers a range of in-house fertility, gynaecological, obstetric and
diagnostic services. The Hospital provides 24-hour nursing services.
A satellite/transport IVF service operates at the North East London
Fertility Centre in Ilford.

London Gynaecology & Fertility Centre

Cozens House
112a Harley Street
London
W1G 7JH

PHONE: 020 7224 0707
Clinical Director: Professor Ian
Craft

(NHS) (SF) (£R) (🚐) (🍼) (24)

TREATMENTS AND SERVICES
IVF, ICSI, GIFT, SO/IUI, DI, IVF w/donor, GIFT w/donor, egg donation,
sperm recovery, tubal surgery, assisted hatching, embryo store, sperm
store, egg store, frozen embryo replacement, sperm donation, embryo
donation, ZIFT

ELIGIBILITY CRITERIA
F 55yrs max, smokers encouraged to stop

ONE CYCLE OF IVF £2550
Not included some/all: blood tests, screening tests, counselling, drugs

ONE CYCLE OF IUI W/DONOR £700 (1 INSEMINATION – 2 INSEMINATIONS £800)
Not included some/all: blood tests, screening tests, counselling, drugs,
sperm sample (£150)

WAITING TIMES IN WEEKS	NHS	PRIVATE
For initial consultation	2	2
To start treatment IVF	0	0
To start treatment IUI w/donor sperm	0	0

DIAGNOSTIC TESTS ACCEPTED
semen analysis, biochemistry, HIV screen (tests results must be recent)

SUPPORT SERVICES
independent counselling, independent support group, talks with previous
patients can be arranged

STAFFING
one physician throughout, dedicated counsellor

CONSULTANTS
Dr Rami Al-Nasser, Dr Anna Carby, Professor Ian Craft, Dr Ehab Kelada,
Dr Marika Mikola, Dr Geetha Venkataraman

The London Gynaecology & Fertility Centre offers a full range of
specialist fertility investigations, treatments and obstetric care under one
roof. The Centre is led by Professor Ian Craft, whose team was responsible for Europe's first IVF twins in 1982. The centre received the first UK
ICSI licence, and pioneered sperm retrieval by needle aspiration (PESA)
and testicular sperm aspiration (TESA) for men with absent vas deferens
or failed vasectomy reversal. There are 3 full-time egg-donor recruiting
staff within the Logan Centre department.

London Women's Clinic

113–115 Harley Street
London
W1N 1DG

PHONE: 020 7487 5050
Medical Consultant: Ms Jinan Bekir
(1968)

(SF) (£R) (🚐) (🧴)

TREATMENTS AND SERVICES
IVF, ICSI, SO/IUI, DI, IVF w/donor, egg donation, egg sharing, sperm recovery, assisted hatching, embryo store, sperm store, blastocyst embryo transfer, IVF surrogacy

ELIGIBILITY CRITERIA
F 46yrs max (50yrs w/donated eggs), BMI< 30, relationship 6 months min, patients should agree to GP's involvement, smokers advised to stop

ONE CYCLE OF IVF £2100
Not included some/all: consultations, screening tests, HFEA fee, drugs

ONE CYCLE OF IUI W/DONOR £490 (WITHOUT SCANS £325)
Not included some/all: consultations, blood tests, screening tests, HFEA fee, drugs

WAITING TIMES IN WEEKS	NHS	PRIVATE
For initial consultation	n/a	2
To start treatment IVF	n/a	4
To start treatment IUI w/donor sperm	n/a	7

DIAGNOSTIC TESTS ACCEPTED
biochemistry, HIV screen, HVS, chlamydia, Hep B/C, cervical smear, CMV IgG & IgM

SUPPORT SERVICES
independent counselling, advice nurse available 9–5

STAFFING
named nurse system sometimes in operation, dedicated counsellor, one physician for any consultation, but not for scans or egg retrieval

CONSULTANTS
Miss Rina Agrawal (1985), Ms Jinan Bekir (1968), Dr Sanjula Sharma (1986)

The London Women's Clinic (previously the Hallam Medical Centre) has been involved in women's healthcare for over 20 years. The clinic was one of the first infertility centres in the UK to make IVF an 'outpatient procedure' and will accept single women and lesbian couples for treatment. A satellite IVF service is available using BUPA Hospital, Hastings, and Nuffield Hospital, Bournemouth. Patients are encouraged to sign disclosure consent forms in order that the clinic may liaise with their GPs.

Maidstone Fertility Centre

Kent Medical Imaging
60 Churchill Square
King's Hill, West Malling
Kent ME19 4DU

PHONE: 01732 529 643
Clinical Director: Professor Ian
Craft

(NHS) (SF) (£R) (🚗) (👤) (24)

TREATMENTS AND SERVICES (CARRIED OUT AT THE MAIN LONDON CLINIC)
IVF, ICSI, GIFT, SO/IUI, DI, IVF w/donor, GIFT w/donor, egg donation, sperm recovery, tubal surgery, assisted hatching, embryo store, sperm store, egg store, frozen embryo replacement, egg freezing, sperm donation, embryo donation and ZIFT

ELIGIBILITY CRITERIA
F 55yrs max, smokers encouraged to stop

ONE CYCLE OF IVF £1800
Not included some/all: blood tests, screening tests, counselling, drugs

ONE CYCLE OF IUI W/DONOR £650 (1 INSEMINATION – 2 INSEMINATIONS £700)
Not included some/all: blood tests, counselling, screening tests, drugs

---

WAITING TIMES IN WEEKS	NHS	PRIVATE
For initial consultation	2	2
To start treatment IVF	0	0
To start treatment IUI w/donor sperm	0	0

DIAGNOSTIC TESTS ACCEPTED
semen analysis, biochemistry, HIV screen (all accepted if recent)

SUPPORT SERVICES
independent counselling, independent support group, talks with previous patients can be arranged

STAFFING
one physician throughout, dedicated counsellor

CONSULTANTS
Professor Ian Craft, Dr Geetha Venkat

The Maidstone Fertility Centre is part of the London Gynaecology & Fertility Centre and is situated in West Malling. It aims to provide a comprehensive and flexible service using the latest techniques, including the use of lasers. Treatment is consultant led, and the Centre has 3 full-time egg donor recruiting staff at the Logan Centre (within the London Fertility Centre). A satellite/transport IVF service operates at Portsmouth and Chichester.

Manchester Fertility Services

Manchester BUPA Hospital
Russell House, Russell Road
Whalley Range
Manchester M16 8AJ

PHONE: 0161 862 9567
Clinical Director: Dr Brian A
Lieberman (1965)

SF **£R** **👜** **24**

TREATMENTS AND SERVICES
IVF, ICSI, GIFT, IUI, DI, IVF w/donor, egg donation, sperm recovery,
assisted hatching, embryo store, sperm store

ELIGIBILITY CRITERIA
F 50yrs max, BMI<30

ONE CYCLE OF IVF £1990
Not included some/all: drugs
Included: egg recovery under general anaesthesia

ONE CYCLE OF IUI W/DONOR £420
Not included some/all: drugs

WAITING TIMES IN WEEKS	NHS	PRIVATE
For initial consultation	n/a	2
To start treatment IVF	n/a	4
To start treatment IUI w/donor sperm	n/a	4

DIAGNOSTIC TESTS ACCEPTED
semen analysis, biochemistry, HIV screen

SUPPORT SERVICES
independent counselling, independent support group

STAFFING
one physician throughout, dedicated counsellor

CONSULTANTS
Dr Susan A Hotchkies (1984), Dr Rosemary Howell (1981), Dr Brian A
Lieberman (1965), Mr A M Nysenbaum (1977), Dr Elizabeth H E Pease
(1972), Dr Andrew Pickersgill (1989), Dr David W Polson (1980)

Manchester Fertility Services was established in 1986. The clinic provides
patients with clear information about what they offer in terms of
treatment, support, advice and commitment. It offers postgraduate
lectures to assist the education of local GPs. A research licence is held for
in vitro development/implantation of normal human pre-implantation
embryos, compared with uni- or poly-pronucleate pre-embryos.

Middle England Fertility Centre

BUPA Hospital Leicester
Gartree Road
Oadby
Leicester LE2 2FF

PHONE: 0116 265 3023
Clinical Director: Mr Roger
Neuberg (1965)

(SF) (£R) (🍼) (24)

TREATMENTS AND SERVICES
IVF, ICSI, GIFT, SO/IUI, DI, IVF w/donor, GIFT w/donor, egg donation, egg sharing, sperm recovery, tubal surgery, assisted hatching, embryo store, sperm store, sterilisation reversal programme

ELIGIBILITY CRITERIA
F 49yrs max, M 70yrs max, stable relationship 2yrs min, number of previous cycles/maternal weight also considered

ONE CYCLE OF IVF £1900
Not included some/all: consultations, blood tests, screening tests, drugs

ONE CYCLE OF IUI W/DONOR £400 WITH CLOMID (£500 WITH GONADOTROPHINS)
Not included some/all: consultations, blood tests, drugs

WAITING TIMES IN WEEKS	NHS	PRIVATE
For initial consultation	n/a	2
To start treatment IVF	n/a	6
To start treatment IUI w/donor sperm	n/a	4

DIAGNOSTIC TESTS ACCEPTED
semen analysis, biochemistry, HIV screen, hormone profile if performed in first 2 days of cycle, Hepatitis B/C screen

SUPPORT SERVICES
independent counselling, independent support group, free consultation with nurse specialist

STAFFING
one physician throughout, named nurse system, dedicated counsellor

CONSULTANTS
Mr Allan Davidson (1968) (co-medical director), Mr Roger Neuberg (1965)

Established in 1990, the infertility clinic at the BUPA Hospital Leicester treats couples from all over the UK. Specially trained fertility nurses offer support and encouragement during treatment. Initial counselling is offered free of charge. The clinic does not discriminate against any group in society and all requests for treatment are considered on their own merits. Focus is placed on the patient being in control of treatment, the clinic's role being to discuss options and carry out the required treatments, and there is never an obligation to continue with a treatment plan. The clinic runs postgraduate evening meetings for GPs and the infertility nurse specialist meets regularly with practice managers.

Midland Fertility Services

3rd Floor, Centre House
Court Parade
Aldridge
West Midlands WS9 8LT

PHONE: 01922 455 911
Clinical Director: Dr Gillian
Lockwood (1986)

(NHS) (SF) ($R) (car) (person) (24)

TREATMENTS AND SERVICES
IVF, ICSI, SO/IUI, DI, IVF w/donor, egg donation, egg sharing, sperm
recovery, assisted hatching, embryo store, sperm store, egg store, oocyte
freezing, embryo donation, ovarian reserve testing, HyCoSy testing

ELIGIBILITY CRITERIA
advice given to women with raised BMI, morbidly obese women may be
excluded on medical grounds (private patients only)

ONE CYCLE OF IVF £1500
Not included some/all: initial consultation and counselling (additional
£170), HFEA fee, drugs *Included:* embryo freezing/1st year's storage

ONE CYCLE OF IUI W/DONOR £330
Not included some/all: initial consultation and counselling (additional
£170), HFEA fee, drugs, donor sperm (additional £75)

WAITING TIMES IN WEEKS	NHS	PRIVATE
For initial consultation	4	4
To start treatment IVF	4	4
To start treatment IUI w/donor sperm	0	0

DIAGNOSTIC TESTS ACCEPTED
biochemistry, HIV screen, tubal patency test

SUPPORT SERVICES
independent counselling, acupuncture, hypnotic relaxation, stress
management

STAFFING
named nurse system, dedicated counsellor

CONSULTANTS
Dr Peter Bromwich, Dr Gillian Lockwood (1986)

Opened in 1987, Midland Fertility Services is the ninth largest fertility
centre in the country and the only one assessed to BS/ISO quality
standard 9002. Approximately one-third of its patients are NHS funded.
The clinic can provide specialist endocrinology and andrology diagnostic
services. All treatments are carried out on-site and treatment programmes
are designed to keep the number of appointments to a minimum.
Patients from all over the world have received treatment at the clinic
and it has experience of 'shared care' programmes for overseas visitors.
Satellite/transport IVF services are offered in Shrewsbury, with a second
site run by MFS staff at Newcross Hospital in Wolverhampton. GPs are
informed of the progress and outcome of all treatment cycles.

North East London Fertility Services

40 Cameron Road
Seven Kings
Ilford
Essex IG3 8LF

PHONE: 020 8597 7414
Clinical Director: Dr M Segal
(1971)

SF **£R** 🚐 🔋 **24**

TREATMENTS AND SERVICES
IVF, ICSI, GIFT, SO/IUI, DI, IVF w/donor, GIFT w/donor, sperm recovery, sperm store

ELIGIBILITY CRITERIA
subject to individual assessment

ONE CYCLE OF IVF £1700
Not included some/all: screening tests, counselling, HFEA fee, drugs

ONE CYCLE OF IUI W/DONOR £425
Not included some/all: consultations, blood tests, screening tests, HFEA fee, drugs

WAITING TIMES IN WEEKS	NHS	PRIVATE
For initial consultation	n/a	0
To start treatment IVF	n/a	0
To start treatment IUI w/donor sperm	n/a	0

DIAGNOSTIC TESTS ACCEPTED
biochemistry, HIV screen

SUPPORT SERVICES
independent counselling, independent support group

STAFFING
one physician throughout, named nurse system, dedicated counsellor

CONSULTANTS
Dr M Segal (1971)

North East London Fertility Services is a small clinic with a focus on low-technology treatment, but using the satellite facility all types of treatment can be provided. Patients are accepted for initial consultation irrespective of their marital status or sexual preference – clinic policy is that everyone is entitled to an opportunity to discuss their problem. Patient information is available on their website and in leaflet form. A satellite/transport IVF service operates at the London Male and Female Fertility Centre.

North Staffordshire Nuffield Hospital

Assisted Conception Unit
Clayton Road
Newcastle under Lyme
Staffordshire ST5 4DB

PHONE: 01782 382 500
Clinical Director: Mr Manjit Obhrai

SF **£** **®** **⚱** **24**

TREATMENTS AND SERVICES
IVF, ICSI, SO/IUI, DI, IVF w/donor, sperm recovery, tubal surgery, assisted
hatching, embryo store, sperm store, sperm storage prior to
vasectomy/chemotherapy

ELIGIBILITY CRITERIA
F 45yrs max

ONE CYCLE OF IVF £1950
Not included some/all: consultations, blood tests, screening tests, drugs

ONE CYCLE OF IUI W/DONOR £500
Not included some/all: consultations, blood tests, screening tests, drugs

WAITING TIMES IN WEEKS	NHS	PRIVATE
For initial consultation	n/a	0
To start treatment IVF	n/a	0
To start treatment IUI w/donor sperm	n/a	0

DIAGNOSTIC TESTS ACCEPTED
biochemistry, HIV screen

SUPPORT SERVICES
independent counselling, independent support group

STAFFING
named nurse system, dedicated counsellor, patients see 1 of 2 physicians

CONSULTANTS
Mr V Menon, Mr Manjit Obhrai

The clinic has not provided any further information about its services.

NURTURE

Floor B, East Block
Queen's Medical Centre
Nottingham
NG7 2UH

PHONE: 0115 970 9490
Clinical Director: Dr Rahnuma
Kazem (1983)

(NHS) (SF) (£R) (👤) (24)

TREATMENTS AND SERVICES
IVF, ICSI, GIFT, SO/IUI, DI, IVF w/donor, GIFT w/donor, egg donation,
egg sharing, sperm recovery, assisted hatching, embryo store, sperm
store, egg store, ovarian tissue storage

ELIGIBILITY CRITERIA
subject to individual assessment

ONE CYCLE OF IVF £2300
Not included some/all: screening tests *Included:* monitoring, counselling,
embryo freezing if required, general anaesthetic for egg collection

ONE CYCLE OF IUI W/DONOR £575
Not included some/all: screening tests, drugs
Included: unlimited counselling

WAITING TIMES IN WEEKS	NHS	PRIVATE
For initial consultation	8	8
To start treatment IVF	0	0
To start treatment IUI w/donor sperm	0	0

DIAGNOSTIC TESTS ACCEPTED
biochemistry, HIV screen, Hepatitis B/C, VDRL/ TRHA, cystic fibrosis

SUPPORT SERVICES
independent counselling, independent support group, occasional stress
management workshops and adoption information evenings

STAFFING
dedicated counsellor

CONSULTANTS
Dr Majeed Aloum, Dr Rahnuma Kazem (1983), Dr David Morroll (1985)

NURTURE was established in 1991and has a team of over 30 doctors,
nurses, scientists and support staff. Its egg share scheme can provide
treatment at reduced cost to patients willing to share their eggs with
other couples. The unit aims to develop new options for diagnosis and
treatment and is currently examining the use of 3D ultrasound to investigate blood flow in the ovaries and uterus, as well as improving methods
of freezing eggs and embryos. It retains close ties with its patients and in
2001 celebrated a decade of treatment, coinciding with the birth of its
2000th baby. Postgraduate information events are organised for GPs
and a research licence is held for egg maturation/cryopreservation and
vitrification of human eggs and embryos.

Oxford Fertility Unit

Level 4, Women's Centre
John Radcliffe Hospital
Headington
Oxford OX3 9DU

PHONE: 01865 221 900
Clinical Director: Mr Enda McVeigh

NHS SF ®£ 🚐 💊 24

TREATMENTS AND SERVICES
IVF, ICSI, SO/IUI, DI, IVF w/donor, egg donation, sperm recovery, tubal
surgery, embryo store, sperm store, blastocyst transfer

ELIGIBILITY CRITERIA
subject to individual assessment

ONE CYCLE OF IVF £1486
Not included some/all: drugs

ONE CYCLE OF IUI W/DONOR £-
Not included some/all: -

WAITING TIMES IN WEEKS	NHS	PRIVATE
For initial consultation	-	-
To start treatment IVF	-	-
To start treatment IUI w/donor sperm	-	-

DIAGNOSTIC TESTS ACCEPTED
biochemistry, HIV screen, lap and dye tests

SUPPORT SERVICES
independent counselling, independent support group, information
evenings, presentations for new patients

STAFFING
named nurse system, dedicated counsellor

CONSULTANTS
Professor D Barlow, Mr Stephen Kennedy, Mr Enda McVeigh

Oxford Fertility Unit was established in 1985 and is staffed by a multi-
disciplinary team. In addition to the range of treatments on offer, the
unit has its own andrology laboratory where tests are undertaken to
investigate male infertility. The unit is run on a non-profit-making basis,
keeping costs as low as possible. It is recognised that every couple
visiting the clinic is different and they will be offered the opportunity
to discuss their own individual circumstances and needs with staff.
A satellite/transport service is available. Liaison with local GPs includes
information mail-shots and presentations.

Peninsular Centre for Repro. Medicine

Exeter Fertility Clinic
Heavitree Hospital
Gladstone Road
Exeter EX1 2ED

PHONE: 01392 405 051
Clinical Director: Mr Jonathan H
West (1978)

(NHS) (SF) (£) (R£) (🚑) (💊) (24)

TREATMENTS AND SERVICES
IVF, ICSI, SO/IUI, DI, IVF w/donor, egg donation, egg sharing, sperm
recovery, tubal surgery, embryo store, sperm store, blastocyst culture,
known donation

ELIGIBILITY CRITERIA
F 50yrs max, M 60yrs max, minimum 1yr relationship, BMI within normal
range

ONE CYCLE OF IVF £1868
Not included some/all: consultations, blood tests, screening tests,
counselling, drugs

ONE CYCLE OF IUI W/DONOR £370
Not included some/all: consultations, blood tests, screening tests, drugs

WAITING TIMES IN WEEKS	NHS	PRIVATE
For initial consultation	24	0
To start treatment IVF	n/a	12
To start treatment IUI w/donor sperm	52	0

DIAGNOSTIC TESTS ACCEPTED
semen analysis, biochemistry, HIV screen

SUPPORT SERVICES
independent counselling, access to nursing staff if required

STAFFING
one physician throughout, named nurse system, dedicated counsellor,
nurse-led care for DI and SO/IUI treatments

CONSULTANTS
Mr Jonathan H West (1978)

The Clinic's philosophy is that all staff support the couple through
investigation, treatment and conclusion. As far as possible, staff are
available to patients and try to ensure that their understanding is
sufficient enough to help inform patient decisions. It is hoped that in this
way patients are able to discuss any fears, anxieties or doubts that they
may have. The Clinic has a 'no baby – no fee' policy. Satellite/transport
IVF service operates at Torbay. GPs have access to patient results via an
encrypted web-page.

Peterborough District Hospital

Fertility Unit
Thorpe Road
Peterborough
Cambridgeshire PE3 6DA

PHONE: 01733 874 516
Clinical Director: Mr John M
Randall (1980)

NHS

TREATMENTS AND SERVICES
DI, tubal surgery, sperm store, full diagnostic service, ovulation induction treatment using injection or pump gonadotrophins, ablation of endometriosis, Clomiphene treatment

ELIGIBILITY CRITERIA
age, number of previous cycles and female weight all inform clinical decision to treat

ONE CYCLE OF IVF £ N/A
Not included some/all: n/a

ONE CYCLE OF IUI W/DONOR £ N/A
Not included some/all: n/a

WAITING TIMES IN WEEKS	NHS	PRIVATE
For initial consultation	12	n/a
To start treatment IVF	n/a	n/a
To start treatment IUI w/donor sperm	n/a	n/a

DIAGNOSTIC TESTS ACCEPTED
semen analysis, biochemistry, HIV screen

SUPPORT SERVICES
independent counselling, 24hr contact number for results, advice and support

STAFFING
one physician throughout, named nurse system, dedicated counsellor

CONSULTANTS
Mr John M Randall (1980)

This is a large dedicated fertility clinic set in an NHS hospital, offering a full range of diagnostic tests. Currently, there is a wait of approximately 2 months for an appointment with the specialist fertility sister or consultant. The clinic offers hour-long initial consultations to take medical histories, give preconceptual health advice and answer any questions. As *some* treatments are not available on the NHS in this area, the clinic tries to refer couples needing private treatment to a unit in the area that best suits their individual needs, and will offer tests needed beforehand and consultations to discuss assisted conception treatments in depth.

Queen Elizabeth Hospital

Centre for Reproductive Medicine
Sheriff Hill
Gateshead
Tyne and Wear NE9 6SX

PHONE: 0191 403 2768
Clinical Director: Mr Ian Aird
(1987)

(NHS) (SF) (£R) (🍾)

TREATMENTS AND SERVICES
IVF, ICSI, SO/IUI, DI, IVF w/donor, egg donation on known donor basis, embryo store, sperm store

ELIGIBILITY CRITERIA
subject to individual assessment

ONE CYCLE OF IVF £1300
Not included some/all: drugs

ONE CYCLE OF IUI W/DONOR £350
Not included some/all: drugs

WAITING TIMES IN WEEKS	NHS	PRIVATE
For initial consultation	3	3
To start treatment IVF	80	12
To start treatment IUI w/donor sperm	16	12

DIAGNOSTIC TESTS ACCEPTED
semen analysis, biochemistry, HIV screen

SUPPORT SERVICES
independent counselling, consultant available 24hrs/7 days a week for emergencies

STAFFING
one physician throughout, named nurse system, dedicated counsellor

CONSULTANTS
Mr Ian Aird (1987)

The Centre for Assisted Reproduction is a self-contained unit within the Queen Elizabeth Hospital offering a range of fertility treatments to both NHS and self-funded patients. Their team of specialists aims to provide a personalised approach to patient care whilst maintaining patient privacy and individuality. The centre offers evening seminars to GPs once or twice a year. A research licence is held for the expression of Trophinin, Tastin and Bystin complex in embryo-indometrial interaction.

Queen Mary's Hospital

Fertility Unit
Frognal Avenue
Sidcup
Kent DA14 6LT

PHONE: 020 8308 3043
Clinical Director: Miss L S Hanna
(1976)

TREATMENTS AND SERVICES
IVF, ICSI, SO/IUI, DI, IVF w/donor, tubal surgery, laparoscopic surgery

ELIGIBILITY CRITERIA
F 45yrs max, NHS patients meeting criteria receive 1 fully funded
treatment

ONE CYCLE OF IVF £800
Not included some/all: drugs

ONE CYCLE OF IUI W/DONOR £250
Not included some/all: drugs, donor sperm sample (additional £125)

WAITING TIMES IN WEEKS	NHS	PRIVATE
For initial consultation	24	24
To start treatment IVF	36	36
To start treatment IUI w/donor sperm	8	8

DIAGNOSTIC TESTS ACCEPTED
semen analysis, biochemistry, HIV screen

SUPPORT SERVICES
independent counselling, independent support group

STAFFING
one physician throughout, dedicated counsellor

CONSULTANTS
Miss L S Hanna (1976)

The Fertility Unit at Queen Mary's Hospital provides treatment to NHS
patients under set funding criteria. Some couples will receive 1 fully
funded treatment cycle (including drugs) plus 2 self-funded cycles.
Others will receive up to 3 self-funded cycles. A satellite/transport IVF
service is available at Chelsfield Park Hospital.

Shropshire & Mid-Wales Fertility Centre

Royal Shrewsbury Hospital
Mytton Oak Road
Shrewsbury
Shropshire SY3 8XQ

PHONE: 01743 261 202
Clinical Director: Mr B Bentick
(1978)

(NHS) (SF) (£R)

TREATMENTS AND SERVICES
IVF, ICSI, SO/IUI, DI, sperm recovery, tubal surgery, embryo store, sperm store

ELIGIBILITY CRITERIA
no previous children including adopted

ONE CYCLE OF IVF £1500
Not included some/all: counselling, drugs

ONE CYCLE OF IUI W/DONOR £611
Not included some/all: n/a

WAITING TIMES IN WEEKS	NHS	PRIVATE
For initial consultation	12	0
To start treatment IVF	156	0
To start treatment IUI w/donor sperm	24	0

DIAGNOSTIC TESTS ACCEPTED
biochemistry, HIV screen

SUPPORT SERVICES
independent counselling, independent support group

STAFFING
one physician throughout, dedicated counsellor

CONSULTANTS
Mr B Bentick (1978)

The Shropshire & Mid-Wales Fertility Centre prides itself on the quality of care offered to its patients, both private and NHS. The small team of nurses, specialist clinical scientists and counsellor are always available for advice and support. Treatment is based on a multi-disciplinary approach. Patients requiring information can call for an informal chat.

Southmead Hospital

Fertility Unit
Cotswold Women's Centre
Bristol
BS10 5NB

PHONE: 0117 959 5102
Clinical Director: Mr Peter Wardle
(1975)

TREATMENTS AND SERVICES
IVF, SO/IUI, DI, egg donation, tubal surgery, embryo store, sperm store

ELIGIBILITY CRITERIA
F 45yrs max, M 60yrs max, 1 child max for IVF/3 children for other treatments, heterosexual couples only, must be married for DI/egg donation, 2yr relationship min, max 4 previous cycles for IUI, 3 previous for IVF, 15 previous for DI, BMI <35 for stimulated cycles, no smokers for IVF

ONE CYCLE OF IVF £ N/A
Not included some/all: n/a

ONE CYCLE OF IUI W/DONOR £ N/A
Not included some/all: n/a

WAITING TIMES IN WEEKS	NHS	PRIVATE
For initial consultation	32	n/a
To start treatment IVF	164	n/a
To start treatment IUI w/*partner's* sperm	32	n/a

DIAGNOSTIC TESTS ACCEPTED
biochemistry, HIV screen, semen analysis if carried out at recognised laboratory

SUPPORT SERVICES
independent counselling

STAFFING
one physician throughout, dedicated counsellor

CONSULTANTS
Mr Peter Wardle (1975)

This NHS clinic provides services to local Health Authority residents. Approximately 700 new couples are seen each year. The clinic also provides an annual study day for local GPs.

South West Centre for Repro. Medicine

Department of Obstetrics
& Gynaecology, Level 06
Derriford Hospital
Plymouth PL6 8DH

PHONE: 01752 763 704
Clinical Director: Dr Umesh
Acharya (1983)

SF **®R** **🚐** **👤**

TREATMENTS AND SERVICES
IVF, ICSI, SO/IUI, DI, IVF w/donor, egg donation, sperm recovery, tubal
surgery, assisted hatching, embryo store, sperm store

ELIGIBILITY CRITERIA
subject to individual assessment

ONE CYCLE OF IVF £1850 (UNDER REVIEW)
Not included some/all: consultations, blood tests, screening tests, HFEA
fee, drugs

ONE CYCLE OF IUI W/DONOR £200 (UNDER REVIEW)
Not included some/all: consultations, blood tests, screening tests, drugs

WAITING TIMES IN WEEKS	NHS	PRIVATE
For initial consultation	n/a	0
To start treatment IVF	n/a	0
To start treatment IUI w/*partner's* sperm	n/a	0

DIAGNOSTIC TESTS ACCEPTED
semen analysis, biochemistry, HIV screen

SUPPORT SERVICES
independent counselling, independent support group

STAFFING
one physician throughout, dedicated counsellor

CONSULTANTS
Dr Umesh Acharya (1983)

The Centre is located within the Ocean Suite in the east wing of
Derriford Hospital. It serves both the local population and patients from
further afield and is a non-profit-making clinic. Three doctors work
within the department together with 5 nurses, 3 clerical staff,
embryologists and a counsellor who is available to patients at any stage
of their investigation or treatment. The clinic provides organised talks
about fertility and assisted conception for GPs, and runs a satellite/
transport IVF service with Torbay.

St James's University Hospital, Leeds

Assisted Conception Unit
Beckett Street
Leeds
LS9 7TF

PHONE: 0113 206 5387
Clinical Director: Mrs Vinay
Sharma (1976)

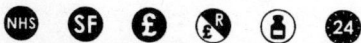

(NHS) (SF) (£) (£R) (bottle) (24)

TREATMENTS AND SERVICES
IVF, ICSI, SO/IUI, DI, IVF w/donor, egg donation, sperm recovery, tubal
surgery, embryo store, sperm store, egg store

ELIGIBILITY CRITERIA
F 45yrs max, M 55yrs max, relationship 1yr min, BMI must not be higher
than 35–40

ONE CYCLE OF IVF £1890
Not included some/all: blood tests, screening tests, drugs

ONE CYCLE OF IUI W/DONOR £360
Not included some/all: drugs

WAITING TIMES IN WEEKS	NHS	PRIVATE
For initial consultation	12	3
To start treatment IVF	0	0
To start treatment IUI w/donor sperm	0	0

DIAGNOSTIC TESTS ACCEPTED
biochemistry and HIV screen accepted, semen analysis and pelvic scan
are always repeated

SUPPORT SERVICES
independent counselling, independent support group, access to staff 7
days a week

STAFFING
one physician throughout, dedicated counsellor

CONSULTANTS
Mrs Vinay Sharma (1976)

This NHS service places emphasis on cost-effectiveness, inclusiveness
and minimally invasive procedures. Patients are guided through
decisions about the continuation of treatment. There is constant
consultant presence and supervision with easy access to staff for advice.
The clinic has robust risk-assessment as well as quality assurance and
assessment protocols. The clinic is a part of an MRC Co-op conducting
research on human embryos.

St Jude's Clinic for Fertility & Gynaecology

The White House
194 Penn Road
Wolverhampton
West Midlands WV3 0EQ

PHONE: 01902 620 831
Clinical Director: Mr Jude Adeghe
(1980)

(NHS) (SF) (£R) (♀) (24)

TREATMENTS AND SERVICES
IVF, ICSI, SO/IUI, DI, IVF w/donor, sperm recovery, tubal surgery, embryo
store, sperm store, Fallopian tube sperm perfusion, surrogacy

ELIGIBILITY CRITERIA
F 50yrs max

ONE CYCLE OF IVF £1600
Not included some/all: drugs

ONE CYCLE OF IUI W/DONOR £500
Not included some/all: drugs

WAITING TIMES IN WEEKS	NHS	PRIVATE
For initial consultation	0	0
To start treatment IVF	0	0
To start treatment IUI w/donor sperm	0	0

DIAGNOSTIC TESTS ACCEPTED
semen analysis, biochemistry, HIV screen

SUPPORT SERVICES
independent counselling, independent support group

STAFFING
one physician throughout, dedicated counsellor, flexible appointments
system

CONSULTANTS
Mr Jude Adeghe (1980)

The Clinic's mission statement is to provide 'individualised quality care
for women and couples'. It offers a friendly environment with flexible
appointments. The dedicated team of doctors, nurses, scientists and
administrative staff are all highly qualified and experienced in the field
of infertility.

Sunderland Fertility Centre

Sunderland Royal Hospital
Kayll Road
Sunderland
Tyne and Wear SR3 1AA

PHONE: 0191 569 9166
Clinical Director: Miss M Dalton
(1975)

TREATMENTS AND SERVICES
SO/IUI, DI, sperm store

ELIGIBILITY CRITERIA
criteria depends on the NHS area in which the patient resides

ONE CYCLE OF IVF £ N/A
Not included some/all: n/a

ONE CYCLE OF IUI W/DONOR £ N/A
Not included some/all: n/a

WAITING TIMES IN WEEKS	NHS	PRIVATE
For initial consultation	8	n/a
To start treatment IVF	n/a	n/a
To start treatment IUI w/donor sperm	8	n/a

DIAGNOSTIC TESTS ACCEPTED
biochemistry

SUPPORT SERVICES
independent counselling

STAFFING
one physician throughout, dedicated counsellor

CONSULTANTS
Miss M Dalton (1975)

The Sunderland Fertility Centre is an NHS secondary fertility clinic, working to provide a wide range of services to help couples with infertility problems. Despite limited resources, the staff are very committed to trying to provide a first class service. Local GPs are offered lectures by the Centre's staff.

Thames Valley Nuffield Hospital

Willow
Wexham Street
Wexham
Buckinghamshire SL3 6NH

PHONE: 01753 665 431
Clinical Director: Mr Neale R
Watson (1983)

(SF) (£) (£R) (🍼) (24)

TREATMENTS AND SERVICES
IVF, ICSI, GIFT, SO/IUI, DI, IVF w/donor, GIFT w/donor, egg donation,
sperm recovery, tubal surgery, embryo store, sperm store, awaiting
licence for assisted hatching

ELIGIBILITY CRITERIA
F 45yrs max, relationship 1yr minimum, advice given to smokers, patients
with FSH level over 10 would be advised regarding probable success rate

ONE CYCLE OF IVF £1950
Not included some/all: blood tests, screening tests, drugs
Included: ultrasound scan by consultant, private room, general
anaesthetic and follow-up after failed cycle/antenatal scan

ONE CYCLE OF IUI W/DONOR £560
Not included some/all: blood tests, screening tests, drugs

WAITING TIMES IN WEEKS	NHS	PRIVATE
For initial consultation	n/a	2
To start treatment IVF	n/a	0
To start treatment IUI w/donor sperm	n/a	0

DIAGNOSTIC TESTS ACCEPTED
biochemistry, HIV screen, Hepatitis B/C

SUPPORT SERVICES
independent counselling, independent support group, nurse counsellors

STAFFING
care provided by 1 of 2 physicians, dedicated counsellor, 24-hour on-call
named nurse

CONSULTANTS
Mr Laurence Macarenhas (1986), Mr Jonathan W A Ramsay (1979),
Mr Neale R Watson (1983)

The Willow clinic progressed to a full infertility service over a 2yr period.
Its staff appreciate the difficulties couples face balancing fertility
treatment with work commitments, and life in general. Appointment
times therefore try to accommodate patients' schedules. A dedicated
embryologist is available to the patient at all stages of treatment, and
each couple is offered a 1hr planning session prior to commencement
of the cycle, aimed at reducing stress and anxiety. The clinic also runs
evenings for GPs with talks given by members of the Willow team.

Tower House Clinic

22a Somerset Street
Kingsdown
Bristol
BS2 8LZ

PHONE: 0117 924 7152
Clinical Director: Dr B L Skew

SF **(A)**

TREATMENTS AND SERVICES
DI, sperm store

ELIGIBILITY CRITERIA
F 45yrs max, M 60yrs max, married couples only

ONE CYCLE OF IVF £ N/A
Not included some/all: n/a

ONE CYCLE OF IUI W/DONOR £ N/A
Not included some/all: n/a

WAITING TIMES IN WEEKS	NHS	PRIVATE
For initial consultation	n/a	0
To start treatment IVF	n/a	n/a
To start treatment IUI w/donor sperm	n/a	n/a

DIAGNOSTIC TESTS ACCEPTED
semen analysis, biochemistry, HIV screen

SUPPORT SERVICES
independent counselling

STAFFING
one physician throughout

CONSULTANTS
Dr B L Skew

Tower House is a small clinic offering a personal donor insemination service. Patients have daily access by telephone to the clinic director and clinician who manage all treatment cycles.

University College Hospital

Assisted Conception Unit
Private Patients Wing
25 Grafton Way
London WC1E 6DB

PHONE: 020 7380 9955
Medical Director: Mr Paul Serhal
(1981)

SF **R£** **(b)** **24**

TREATMENTS AND SERVICES
IVF, ICSI, GIFT, SO/IUI, DI, IVF w/donor, GIFT w/donor, egg donation,
egg sharing, sperm recovery, tubal surgery, assisted hatching, embryo
store, sperm store, egg store, PGD

ELIGIBILITY CRITERIA
F 49yrs max, M 70yrs max

ONE CYCLE OF IVF £2250
Not included some/all: consultations, blood tests, screening tests,
counselling, HFEA fee, drugs

ONE CYCLE OF IUI W/DONOR £550
Not included some/all: consultations, blood tests, screening tests,
counselling, HFEA fee, drugs

WAITING TIMES IN WEEKS	NHS*	PRIVATE
For initial consultation	n/a	1
To start treatment IVF	n/a	4
To start treatment IUI w/donor sperm	n/a	0

DIAGNOSTIC TESTS ACCEPTED
semen analysis, biochemistry, HIV screen

SUPPORT SERVICES
independent counselling

STAFFING
one physician throughout, named nurse system

CONSULTANTS
Dr Maurice Katz (1963), Mr Paul Serhal (1981)

The ACU is situated in the Rosenheim Building at University College
London Hospitals. It has offered a comprehensive range of treatments
and investigative procedures since 1990. Collaboration with the genetics
team at University College London has led to the pioneering of new
techniques for Pre-Implantation Genetic Diagnosis, for which a research
licence is held. Initial consultations can usually be arranged within 10
days. Wherever possible, treatment programmes are arranged to suit the
patient's individual requirements.
* NHS patients are occasionally treated at this clinic when specialised
services are required eg egg freezing – NHS waiting times are therefore
not applicable.

University Hospital Aintree

Assisted Conception Clinic
Ward 1A
Lower Lane
Liverpool L9 7AL

PHONE: 0151 529 3800
Clinical Director: Mr Geoffrey
Shaw (1980)

(NHS) (SF) (£R) (🚹) (24)

TREATMENTS AND SERVICES
IVF, ICSI, GIFT, SO/IUI, DI, IVF w/donor, sperm recovery, tubal surgery,
embryo store, sperm store

ELIGIBILITY CRITERIA
NHS patients have to fulfil PCT criteria, private patients subject to
individual assessment

ONE CYCLE OF IVF £2600
Not included some/all: n/a

ONE CYCLE OF IUI W/DONOR £195
Not included some/all: n/a but if gonadotrophins are needed in
treatment, patients pay for these on a pro-rata basis

WAITING TIMES IN WEEKS	NHS	PRIVATE
For initial consultation	8	8
To start treatment IVF	-	8
To start treatment IUI w/donor sperm	-	0

DIAGNOSTIC TESTS ACCEPTED
biochemistry, HIV screen

SUPPORT SERVICES
independent counselling, independent support group

STAFFING
named nurse system, dedicated counsellor

CONSULTANTS
Mr Geoffrey Shaw (1980)

In 1986 a group of patients liaised with University Hospital in Aintree and
raised funds in order to establish the unit, which opened in 1988. It has
maintained strong links with those it was set up to help, and provides
both NHS and self-funded treatments on a non-profit-making basis.
Usually, consultants do not charge fees, even for self-funded treatment.
It was the first infertility unit in the UK to be awarded the government's
Chartermark for excellence in the provision of public service. Based at
University Hospital in Aintree, the Unit has recently become part of the
Liverpool Women's Hospital Trust, one of the largest providers of
infertility treatment in the UK.

Washington Hospital Cromwell IVF & Fertility Unit

BUPA Washington Hospital
Picktree Lane, Rickleton
Washington
Tyne and Wear NE38 9JZ

PHONE: 0191 417 6463
Clinical Director: Mr Eric Simons
(1962)

(NHS) (SF) (£R) (🍼)

TREATMENTS AND SERVICES
IVF, ICSI, SO/IUI, DI, IVF w/donor, egg donation, egg sharing, sperm
recovery, assisted hatching, embryo store, sperm store, blastocyst
transfer, vasectomy reversal

ELIGIBILITY CRITERIA
F 58yrs max, stable heterosexual relationship required, egg donors must
cease smoking 3 months before treatment, weight loss advised if BMI>30

ONE CYCLE OF IVF £2250
Not included some/all: initial consultation, blood tests, screening tests,
HFEA fee

ONE CYCLE OF IUI W/DONOR £535
Not included some/all: initial consultation, blood tests, screening tests,
HFEA fee, drugs (additional £65)

WAITING TIMES IN WEEKS	NHS	PRIVATE
For initial consultation	-	-
To start treatment IVF	-	-
To start treatment IUI w/donor sperm	-	-

DIAGNOSTIC TESTS ACCEPTED
biochemistry, HIV screen, scans

SUPPORT SERVICES
independent counselling, independent support group

STAFFING
one physician throughout, dedicated counsellor

CONSULTANTS
Mr Eric Simons (1962)

The Cromwell IVF Centre at the Washington Hospital pioneered the
concept of egg sharing in the UK, and successfully persuaded the HFEA
to incorporate it into the National Code of Practice. Currently the
programme is one of the largest egg sharing services in Europe.

Watford General Hospital

Fertility Clinic
Vicarage Road
Watford
Hertfordshire WD1 8HB

PHONE: 01923 217 936
Clinical Director: Mr Malloum
Padwick (1980)

NHS (b)

TREATMENTS AND SERVICES
SO/IUI, DI, sperm store

ELIGIBILITY CRITERIA
subject to individual assessment

ONE CYCLE OF IVF £ N/A
Not included some/all: n/a

ONE CYCLE OF IUI W/DONOR £ N/A
Not included some/all: n/a

WAITING TIMES IN WEEKS	NHS	PRIVATE
For initial consultation	-	n/a
To start treatment IVF	-	n/a
To start treatment IUI w/donor sperm	-	n/a

DIAGNOSTIC TESTS ACCEPTED
semen analysis, HIV screen

SUPPORT SERVICES
independent counselling, nurse practitioner available

STAFFING
one physician throughout, named nurse system, dedicated counsellor

CONSULTANTS
Dr A Leahy, Mr Malloum Padwick (1980)

This is a small NHS clinic accepting referrals from GPs and local
gynaecologists. Medical staff assess patients by detailed history taking,
examination and investigation. Nurse practitioners respond to all queries
from patients, perform ultrasound scans, DI and IUI, and provide
informal counselling. Patients also have access to a formal independent
counsellor. Patients are referred to assisted conception units if this is
necessary after assessment.

Wessex Fertility Services/BUPA Chalybeate IVF Unit

Princess Anne Hospital
Coxford Road
Southampton SO16 5YA
PHONE: 023 8076 4318
Clinical Director: Mr G Masson (1968)

BUPA Chalybeate Hospital
Chalybeate Close, Tremona Road
Southampton SO16 6UY
PHONE: 023 8076 4318
Clinical Director: Mr G Masson (1968)

(NHS) (SF) (£R) (🚐) (🍼) (24)

TREATMENTS AND SERVICES
IVF, ICSI, GIFT, SO/IUI, DI, IVF w/donor, egg donation, egg sharing,
sperm recovery, tubal surgery, assisted hatching, embryo store, sperm
store

ELIGIBILITY CRITERIA
previous response, FSH levels and age of female donor recipient
considered

ONE CYCLE OF IVF £2310
Not included some/all: initial consultation, screening tests, initial
hormone profile/infection screens, gonadotrophin

ONE CYCLE OF IUI W/DONOR £330
Not included some/all: initial consultation, scans, blood tests, screening
tests, HFEA fee, drugs

WAITING TIMES IN WEEKS	NHS	PRIVATE
For initial consultation	8	3
To start treatment IVF	0	0
To start treatment IUI w/donor sperm	0	0

DIAGNOSTIC TESTS ACCEPTED
biochemistry, HIV screen

SUPPORT SERVICES
independent counselling, independent support group

STAFFING
dedicated counsellor, small team that attempts to keep same staff
involved throughout a patient's treatment

CONSULTANTS
Mr G Masson (1968)

This clinic was established in 1986 and offers a wide range of services.
GPs are kept informed by letter and the clinic provides a final summary of
treatment. A satellite/transport service is provided in the Channel Islands,
Salisbury and Bournemouth.

West Middlesex University Hospital

Department of Gynaecology
Twickenham Road
Isleworth
Middlesex TW7 6AF

PHONE: 020 8565 5117
Clinical Director: Dr Elizabeth
Owen (1980)

(NHS) (⬤) (24)

TREATMENTS AND SERVICES
SO/IUI, DI, sperm store

ELIGIBILITY CRITERIA
F 42yrs max, 2 previous children max (not incl. adopted), min 1yr relationship if under 35 yrs/6 months min if over 35 yrs, BMI<30, max 4
previous cycles of SO/IUI

ONE CYCLE OF IVF £ N/A
Not included some/all: n/a

ONE CYCLE OF IUI W/DONOR £120
Not included some/all: sperm is obtained from UCL and London
Women's Clinic – this fee covers the cost of this

WAITING TIMES IN WEEKS	NHS	PRIVATE
For initial consultation	8	n/a
To start treatment IVF	n/a	n/a
To start treatment IUI w/donor sperm	0	n/a

DIAGNOSTIC TESTS ACCEPTED
semen analysis, biochemistry

SUPPORT SERVICES
independent counselling, independent support group

STAFFING
one physician throughout, named nurse system

CONSULTANTS
Dr Elizabeth Owen (1980)

The unit at West Middlesex University Hospital offers superovulation
and insemination, and ovulation induction and donor insemination on
the NHS. Patients are seen and treatment decisions made at weekly
infertility clinics. Each patient is offered 4 cycles of superovulation and
insemination, 2 with Clomid, 2 with cl+lmcg. The unit is staffed by
a consultant, staff specialist, infertility nurse and counsellor, with another
consultant dedicated to donor inseminations. Scans and IUIs are carried
out on the same floor as the laboratory, and trained laboratory staff carry
out sperm washing. The unit holds meetings with GPs in the community.

Winterbourne Fertility Centre

The Winterbourne Hospital
Herringston Road
Dorchester
Dorset DT1 2DR

PHONE: 01305 263 252
Clinical Director: Mr Michael
Dooley (1980)

(NHS) (SF) (£) (R£) (🚗) (👤) (24)

TREATMENTS AND SERVICES
IVF, ICSI, GIFT, SO/IUI, DI, IVF w/donor, GIFT w/donor, egg donation,
sperm recovery, tubal surgery, embryo store, sperm store, diet/lifestyle
advice and complementary therapy if needed, advice also given to
smokers

ELIGIBILITY CRITERIA
F 50ys max

ONE CYCLE OF IVF £2490
Not included some/all: initial consultation, screening tests, drugs

ONE CYCLE OF IUI W/DONOR £575
Not included some/all: initial consultation, screening tests, drugs

WAITING TIMES IN WEEKS	NHS	PRIVATE
For initial consultation	-	3
To start treatment IVF	-	4
To start treatment IUI w/donor sperm	-	0

DIAGNOSTIC TESTS ACCEPTED
biochemistry, HIV screen

SUPPORT SERVICES
independent counselling, independent support group

STAFFING
1 physician throughout, 3 nurses, 3 embryologists

CONSULTANTS
Mr Michael Dooley (1980), Mr Julian Pampiglione (1980)

The Winterbourne Fertility Centre aims to provide comprehensive
diagnostic and treatment services to their patients. The centre offers
a holistic approach to treatment, offering advice from other health
professionals in areas such as lifestyle and diet, as well as addressing
the immediate clinical needs of their patients. Satellite IVF services are
provided at The Bournemouth Nuffield and Royal Bournemouth hospitals.

Wirral Fertility Centre

BUPA Murrayfield Hospital
Holmwood Drive
Thingwall, Wirral
Merseyside CH61 1AU

PHONE: 0151 648 2364
Clinical Director: Mr U Abdulla
(1961)

SF ®£ 🚑 🧴 24

TREATMENTS AND SERVICES
IVF, ICSI, SO/IUI, DI, IVF w/donor, tubal surgery, embryo store

ELIGIBILITY CRITERIA
for IVF only: F 40yrs max, couples subject to individual assessment

ONE CYCLE OF IVF £1955
Not included some/all: screening tests, drugs

ONE CYCLE OF IUI W/DONOR £725 (3-CYCLE PACKAGE AVAILABLE AT LOWER COST)
Not included some/all: screening tests, drugs

WAITING TIMES IN WEEKS	NHS	PRIVATE
For initial consultation	n/a	0
To start treatment IVF	n/a	0
To start treatment IUI w/donor sperm	n/a	0

DIAGNOSTIC TESTS ACCEPTED
biochemistry, HIV screen, HSG, lap & dye test

SUPPORT SERVICES
independent counselling, independent support group

STAFFING
dedicated counsellor, 2 physicians, 3 nurses, embryologist

CONSULTANTS
Mr U Abdulla (1961), Mr S A Majid (1970), Mr A Murray (1973)

Since the Wirral Fertility Centre opened in 1990, it has accepted more than 1200 patients. It became fully operational after extensive alterations in 1994. In addition to the wide range of investigations and treatments, the clinic has facilities to freeze embryos and was the first to introduce this technique in Merseyside. Patients' GPs are kept informed of progress throughout treatment.

Woking Nuffield Hospital

Assisted Conception Services
Victoria Wing, Shores Road
Woking
Surrey GU21 4BY

PHONE: 01483 227 859
Clinical Director: Mr Andrew
Riddle (1977)

SF **£** **®** **☺** **24**

TREATMENTS AND SERVICES
IVF, ICSI, GIFT, SO/IUI, DI, IVF w/donor, GIFT w/donor, sperm recovery,
tubal surgery, assisted hatching, embryo store, sperm store

ELIGIBILITY CRITERIA
F 45yrs max, no patients with Hepatitis C or non-treatable terminal
illness, clinical advice given if required on weight or smoking problems

ONE CYCLE OF IVF £2200
Not included some/all: screening tests, drugs
Included: pregnancy test, 6-and 8-week pregnancy scans

ONE CYCLE OF IUI W/DONOR £490
Not included some/all: scans, screening tests, drugs

WAITING TIMES IN WEEKS	NHS	PRIVATE
For initial consultation	n/a	4
To start treatment IVF	n/a	0
To start treatment IUI w/donor sperm	n/a	0

DIAGNOSTIC TESTS ACCEPTED
biochemistry, HIV screen, hormone profiles, chlamydia, CMV, rubella

SUPPORT SERVICES
independent counselling, independent support group

STAFFING
one physician throughout, dedicated counsellor

CONSULTANTS
Mr E P Curtis (1982), Mr Andrew Riddle (1977)

Assisted Conception Services at the Woking Nuffield Hospital is a small
IVF clinic with very experienced staff. Patients can arrange informal visits.

Wolfson Family Clinic/Hammersmith Hospital IVF Unit

Hammersmith Hospital
Du Cane Road
London
W12 0HS

PHONE: 020 8383 4152
Clinical Director: Professor Robert
Winston

(NHS) (SF) (£R) (§) (24)

TREATMENTS AND SERVICES
IVF, ICSI, GIFT, SO/IUI, DI, IVF w/donor, GIFT w/donor, egg donation,
sperm recovery, tubal surgery, assisted hatching, embryo store, sperm
store, comprehensive infertility investigation, PGD, MESA, TESE, blastocyst transfer, FERC (natural & drug cycles), consultant anaesthetic service

ELIGIBILITY CRITERIA
subject to individual assessment

ONE CYCLE OF IVF £1800
Not included some/all: drugs

ONE CYCLE OF IUI W/DONOR £400 (NATURAL CYCLE – STIMULATED £450–£550)
Not included some/all: drugs

WAITING TIMES IN WEEKS	NHS	PRIVATE
For initial consultation	16	1
To start treatment IVF	8	4
To start treatment IUI w/donor sperm	6	6

DIAGNOSTIC TESTS ACCEPTED
all tests performed elsewhere are accepted – investigations only repeated
when necessary

SUPPORT SERVICES
independent counselling

STAFFING
multi-disciplinary team on-site, clinician-led treatment throughout

CONSULTANTS
four full-time consultants including Professor R Winston, Mr R A Margara
and Mr G Trew

Although there is a strong focus on IVF at the Wolfson Family Clinic,
consultants feel that there are many other treatments that may be just as
effective, if not more so. Spacious and comfortable, it has one of the highest staff:patient ratios in Britain with over 50 staff, including 10 doctors.
All tests, investigations, procedures and lab work are undertaken on-site.
Consultant anaesthetist is present for all egg collections, sedations and
general anaesthetics and is offered inclusive of package price. Although
the clinic is a leading British research institute, emphasis is placed on the
emotional care of patients. Occasional open days are held for GPs and
the unit holds a research licence for pre-implantation genetic diagnosis,
genetic defects in embryos and failure of embryonic development.

Wolverhampton Assisted Conception Unit

Directorate of Obstetrics
& Gynaecology, Maternity Unit
New Cross Hospital
Wolverhampton WV10 0QP

PHONE: 01902 642 880
Clinical Director: Dr Gillian
Lockwood (1986)

(NHS) (SF) (£R) (A) (24)

TREATMENTS AND SERVICES
IVF, ICSI, SO/IUI, DI, IVF w/donor, egg donation, egg sharing, sperm recovery, assisted hatching, embryo store, sperm store, egg store, oocyte freezing, embryo donation, HyCoSy tubal patency test, ovarian reserve test

ELIGIBILITY CRITERIA
self-funded patients only; advice given to women with raised BMI, morbidly obese women may be excluded on medical grounds

ONE CYCLE OF IVF £1500
Not included some/all: HFEA fee, drugs (initial counselling and 1st visit are an additional £170) *Included:* embryo freezing/1st year's storage

ONE CYCLE OF IUI W/DONOR £330
Not included some/all: HFEA fee, drugs (initial counselling and first visit costs are additional £170), donor sperm (additional £75)

WAITING TIMES IN WEEKS	NHS	PRIVATE
For initial consultation	2	2
To start treatment IVF	4	4
To start treatment IUI w/donor sperm	0	0

DIAGNOSTIC TESTS ACCEPTED
biochemistry, HIV screen, tubal patency test

SUPPORT SERVICES
independent counselling, acupuncture, hypnotic relaxation, stress management

STAFFING
named nurse system, dedicated counsellor

CONSULTANTS
Dr R Gupta, Dr Gillian Lockwood (1986)

Wolverhampton ACU is a satellite unit of Midland Fertility Services and is situated at New Cross Hospital, close to Wolverhampton town centre. The main clinic is located in a village in Aldridge, just north of Birmingham.

Cardiff Assisted Reproduction Unit

University Hospital of Wales
Heath Park
Cardiff
Wales CF14 4XW

PHONE: 029 2074 2282
Clinical Director: Mr Lukas
Klentzeris (1981)

(NHS) (SF) (®R) (🍼) (24)

TREATMENTS AND SERVICES
IVF, ICSI, SO/IUI, DI, IVF w/donor, egg donation, sperm recovery, tubal
surgery, embryo store, sperm store

ELIGIBILITY CRITERIA
F 50yrs max, M 50yrs max, min 3yr relationship

ONE CYCLE OF IVF £1855
Not included some/all: consultations, drugs

ONE CYCLE OF IUI W/DONOR £505
Not included some/all: consultations, drugs
Included: one follow-up appointment

WAITING TIMES IN WEEKS	NHS	PRIVATE
For initial consultation	32	8
To start treatment IVF	104	12
To start treatment IUI w/donor sperm	104	8

DIAGNOSTIC TESTS ACCEPTED
biochemistry, HIV screen

SUPPORT SERVICES
independent counselling, independent support group

STAFFING
one physician throughout, named nurse system, dedicated counsellor

CONSULTANTS
Mr N M Amso (1979), Mr Lukas Klentzeris (1981)

Established in 1986, CARU is situated in the Women's Unit at the
University Hospital of Wales and is the only unit in Wales to provide
both NHS and self-funded treatment. It operates within an academic
environment and provides a full spectrum of therapeutic options for
couples with fertility problems.

Cromwell IVF & Fertility Centre

Singleton Hospital
Sketty Lane
Swansea
Wales SA2 8QA

PHONE: 01792 285 954
Clinical Director: Mr P Bowen-
Simpkins (1966)

(SF) (£R) (🚐) (👤) (24)

TREATMENTS AND SERVICES
IVF, ICSI, SO/IUI, DI, IVF w/donor, egg donation, egg sharing, sperm
recovery, assisted hatching, embryo store, sperm store

ELIGIBILITY CRITERIA
subject to individual assessment

ONE CYCLE OF IVF £2290
Not included some/all: blood tests, screening tests

ONE CYCLE OF IUI W/DONOR £450
Not included some/all: blood tests, screening tests

WAITING TIMES IN WEEKS	NHS	PRIVATE
For initial consultation	n/a	4
To start treatment IVF	n/a	0
To start treatment IUI w/donor sperm	n/a	0

DIAGNOSTIC TESTS ACCEPTED
no tests performed elsewhere are accepted

SUPPORT SERVICES
independent counselling

STAFFING
one physician throughout, named nurse system, dedicated counsellor

CONSULTANTS
Mr P Bowen-Simpkins (1966), Dr Shailaja Nair (1977), Mr Eric G Simons
(1962)

A satellite/transport IVF service is available at Cardiff BUPA Hospital.

Princess of Wales Hospital

Fertility Clinic
Coity Road
Bridgend
Wales CF31 1RQ

PHONE: 01656 752 465
Lead Clinician: Mr R P Balfour
(1966)

NHS (b)

TREATMENTS AND SERVICES
SO/IUI

ELIGIBILITY CRITERIA
F 42yrs max except IUI where limit is 40yrs, M 60yrs max, 2yr min
relationship for patients under 25yrs, 1yr relationship min for patients
over 30yrs, female weight should be less than 110kg

ONE CYCLE OF IVF £ N/A
Not included some/all: n/a

ONE CYCLE OF IUI W/DONOR £ N/A
Not included some/all: n/a

WAITING TIMES IN WEEKS	NHS	PRIVATE
For initial consultation	8	n/a
To start treatment IVF	n/a	n/a
To start treatment IUI w/donor sperm	n/a	n/a

DIAGNOSTIC TESTS ACCEPTED
semen analysis, biochemistry, HIV screen

SUPPORT SERVICES
miscarriage support

STAFFING
named nurse system

CONSULTANTS
Mr R P Balfour (1966)

This is a small, NHS-funded clinic offering a speedy service. A diagnostic
laparoscopy and dye test can be done within 6 weeks of initial
consultation and facilities exist for laser treatment of endometriosis and
laparoscopic tubular surgery. Patients with PCOS are also offered
laparoscopic surgery. Patients come mainly from the local catchment
area, but GP referrals are accepted from further afield. Reversal of
sterilisation can be carried out on a private basis – this procedure
currently has a 62 per cent success rate.

Glasgow Royal Infirmary

Assisted Conception Unit
Ground Floor, Walton Building
84 Castle Street, Glasgow
Scotland G4 0SF

PHONE: 0141 211 400 ext. 5511
Clinical Director: Dr R W S Yates
(1977)

(NHS) (logo)

TREATMENTS AND SERVICES
IVF, ICSI, SO/IUI, DI, IVF w/donor, egg donation, sperm recovery, tubal
surgery, embryo store, sperm store, ovarian tissue storage facility being
developed

ELIGIBILITY CRITERIA
F 37yrs max, M 55yrs max, previous children must no longer reside with
couple, stable relationship of 2yrs min, BMI<30

ONE CYCLE OF IVF £ N/A
Not included some/all: n/a

ONE CYCLE OF IUI W/DONOR £ N/A
Not included some/all: n/a

WAITING TIMES IN WEEKS	NHS	PRIVATE
For initial consultation	20	n/a
To start treatment IVF	40	n/a
To start treatment IUI w/donor sperm	0	n/a

DIAGNOSTIC TESTS ACCEPTED
no tests performed elsewhere are accepted

SUPPORT SERVICES
independent counselling, independent support group

STAFFING
named nurse system, dedicated counsellor

CONSULTANTS
Dr Helen Lyell, Dr R W S Yates (1977)

The Glasgow Royal Infirmary Assisted Conception Unit is the regional
referral centre for the West of Scotland, providing all aspects of assisted
conception through the NHS. The unit holds a research licence for pre-
implantation genetic diagnosis.

Ninewells Hospital

Assisted Conception Unit
Ninewells Hospital & Medical
School, Dundee
Scotland DD1 9SY

PHONE: 01382 632 111
Clinical Director: Dr Tony Harrold
(1985)

NHS SF £R ⊙ 24

TREATMENTS AND SERVICES
IVF, ICSI, SO/IUI, DI, IVF w/donor, egg donation, sperm recovery, tubal
surgery, assisted hatching, embryo store, sperm store

ELIGIBILITY CRITERIA
relationship 1yr minimum

ONE CYCLE OF IVF £2275
Not included some/all: n/a

ONE CYCLE OF IUI W/DONOR £ N/A
Not included some/all: n/a

WAITING TIMES IN WEEKS	NHS	PRIVATE
For initial consultation	4	4
To start treatment IVF	-	4
To start treatment IUI w/donor sperm	8	n/a

DIAGNOSTIC TESTS ACCEPTED
semen analysis, biochemistry, HIV screen

SUPPORT SERVICES
independent counselling, independent support group

STAFFING
dedicated counsellor

CONSULTANTS
Dr Tony Harrold (1985), Dr John Mills (1966), Dr Rima Rajkohowa (1985)

The Assisted Conception Unit at Ninewells Hospital has been offering
assisted conception treatment since the mid-1980s and has been in its
present location since 1994. It is staffed by a multi-disciplinary team of
medical, nursing, scientific and administrative staff. Approximately 40
per cent of patients at the clinic fund their own treatment.

University of Aberdeen

Assisted Reproduction Unit
Aberdeen Maternity Hospital
Foresterhill, Aberdeen
Scotland AB25 2ZL

PHONE: 01224 554 482
Clinical Director: Dr Mark
Hamilton

NHS **SF** **£R** **(🔋)**

TREATMENTS AND SERVICES
IVF, ICSI, SO/IUI, DI, IVF w/donor, egg donation, sperm recovery, embryo
store, sperm store

ELIGIBILITY CRITERIA
F 45yrs max

ONE CYCLE OF IVF £1750
Not included some/all: drugs

ONE CYCLE OF IUI W/DONOR £350
Not included some/all: drugs

WAITING TIMES IN WEEKS	NHS	PRIVATE
For initial consultation	52	8
To start treatment IVF	4	4
To start treatment IUI w/donor sperm	4	4

DIAGNOSTIC TESTS ACCEPTED
semen analysis, biochemistry

SUPPORT SERVICES
independent counselling, independent support group

STAFFING
named nurse system, dedicated counsellor, appointment with
embryologist if required

CONSULTANTS
Dr Mark Hamilton, Professor Allan A Templeton

Since it opened in 1989, the Assisted Reproduction Unit has been based
in the Department of Obstetrics and Gynaecology at Aberdeen Maternity
Hospital. The unit operates on a non-profit-making basis. Over 500 new
couples are seen every year, and in excess of 600 treatment cycles are
carried out annually. A research licence is held for folate uptake in
embryo development.

Fertility specialist profiles

Mr Hossam Abdalla, Clinical Director – The Lister Hospital ACU
Consultant – Chelsea & Westminster Hospital
Clinical Director of this ACU since 1988, part of his pioneering research led to Britain's first birth from a frozen, thawed, donated embryo which had been transferred to the fallopian tubes using ZIFT. He has also introduced new approaches to ovulation induction and oocyte donation and is a highly experienced laparoscopic surgeon.

Mr Peter Brinsden, Medical Director – Bourn Hall Clinic
After working with Professor Craft as Deputy Director of the Wellington Hospital IVF Unit (then the largest IVF and GIFT Unit in the world), and then with Mr Steptoe at Bourn Hall in 1985, he was appointed Medical Director in 1989. His principal interests are the treatment of male factor infertility (including spinal cord injured men), older infertile women, ovum donation and IVF surrogacy. He is a Fellow of the Royal College of Obstetricians & Gynaecologists.

Professor Ian Craft, Director – London Gynaecology & Fertility
Centre
Upon leaving the professorship of Obstetrics & Gynaecology at the Royal Free Hospital, he set up the London Fertility Centre in 1982. His professorship enabled him to develop his earlier research into the role of fallopian tube environment in human embryo development. His team's pioneering work then resulted in the birth of Europe's first IVF twins in 1982.

Dr Simon Fishel, Director – CARE at The Park Hospital
Working for many years with Professor Edwards, he was part of the team responsible for the world's first test-tube baby in 1978. Elected to the Inspectorate of the HFEA in 1996, he has been Director of CARE at The Park Hospital since 1997. His pioneering work covers the fields of IVF, ICSI, spermatid births, micro-injection technology and ICSI techniques for severe male factor infertility, and he has helped establish fertility clinics worldwide.

Professor J G Grudzinskas, Director – The Bridge Centre
Barts & the London NHS Fertility Centre

After training in Australia, Singapore and London, he became
Professor of Obstetrics & Gynaecology at St Bartholomew's and The
Royal London Hospitals School of Medicine & Dentistry, where he is
also an Honorary Consultant and Senior Examiner. His special
interests include assessment and treatment of infertility linked to
ovarian and tubal function, and risk assessment in early pregnancy.
He has published widely and been awarded an A-standard merit from
the UK's Advisory Committee on Distinction Awards for his
achievements and continuing work for the NHS. He is also a Fellow
of the Royal College of Obstetricians & Gynaecologists.

Mr Julian Jenkins, Clinical Director – Bristol University Centre for
Reproductive Medicine

Clinical Director of the Centre since 1999, he is currently Consultant
Senior Lecturer in Reproductive Medicine at Bristol University. His
particular interest is the application of information technology to
medical practice and his projects have included patient information
systems and clinical decision support tools. A Fellow of the Royal
College of Obstetricians & Gynaecologists and Chairman of the
Obstetrics & Gynaecology education subcommittee for the South
West, he is also a member of various bodies including the Menstrual
Disorder & Infertility Panel of the Cochrane Collaboration.

Mr Charles Kingsland, Clinical Director – Liverpool Women's
Hospital Repro. Medicine Unit, Consultant – Wirral Fertility Centre

In 1989, whilst a lecturer at Liverpool University, he established the
Reproductive Medicine Unit, now the single largest provider of NHS
treatment in the UK. In 1990 he developed the idea of Transport IVF
and created a network with four local hospitals which still runs
today. As a result, Transport IVF is now used all over the UK. He has
published widely on infertility, is an Inspector for the HFEA and a
Fellow of the Royal College of Obstetricians & Gynaecologists.

Dr Gillian Lockwood, Director – Midland Fertility Services

Having qualified first in Philosophy, Politics & Economics and then
in Medicine from Oxford in 1986, she worked at the Oxford Fertility

Unit for ten years researching PCOS, azoospermia and recurrent miscarriage. Director of Midland Fertility Services since 2000, her interest is in the fertility management of women in their '40s and she developed the Inhibin B test for ovarian reserve. Chair of the British Fertility Society Ethics Committee, she lectures and broadcasts regularly on the ethical aspects of assisted reproduction and is on the Editorial Board of 'Human Fertility' and 'Human Reproduction'.

Dr David Morroll, Director – NURTURE

At NURTURE since 1997,he is currently its Director and Senior Clinical Embryologist. He lectures on Nottingham University's MSC course in Assisted Reproductive Technique, and is Chairman of the British Andrology Society Education Committee. Also a member of the Association of Clinical Embryologists Professional Development Committee and Co-ordinator of their Continuing Professional Development programme, he is a Scientific Inspector for the HFEA.

Dr Geeta Nargund, Medical Director – Diana, Princess of Wales Centre for Reproductive Medicine, Associate – Create Health Clinic

Senior Lecturer in Obstetrics & Gynaecology and an Honorary Consultant in Reproductive Medicine at St Georges Hospital Medical School, she pioneered the use of follicular Doppler for egg quality assessment, and 'one-stop' fertility diagnosis using advanced ultra-sound technology, publishing widely on its use in Reproductive Medicine. She also produced the first scientific paper on cumulative live birth rates using Natural Cycle IVF. Her holistic approach aims to establish links between women's reproductive health and life-style/psychological factors. As Chief Executive of the HER TRUST charity, she is committed to helping women help themselves to health.

Mr Anthony Rutherford, Director – Leeds General Infirmary ACU Consultant – BUPA Hospital Leeds, Mid Yorkshire Nuffield Hospital

Since establishing The Clarendon Wing in '91, he has seen the unit grow into one of the largest in the UK. He is an Honorary Senior Lecturer at Leeds General Infirmary with interests in tubal/ minimal access gynaecological surgery, PGD, invitro maturation of oocytes and cryopreservation of ovarian tissue. He is a Fellow of the Royal College of Obstetricians & Gynaecologists and an HFEA Inspector.

Mr Peter Wardle, Clinical Director – Southmead Hospital Fertility Unit, Consultant – Bristol Nuffield at The Chesterfield and St Mary's

Consultant Obstetrician & Gynaecologist and Subspecialist in Reproductive Medicine at Southmead Hospital, he is also a Senior Clinical Lecturer in Obstetrics & Gynaecology at Bristol University. As its former Deputy Head, he maintains links with the University's Centre for Reproductive Medicine. His interests include pubertal disorders, male and female infertility, assisted conception, recurrent miscarriage, gynaecological endocrinology, endometriosis and post-reproductive endocrinology. He is an Inspector for the HFEA and a Fellow of the Royal College of Obstetricians & Gynaecologists.

Professor Robert Winston, Clinical Director – Wolfson Family Clinic/Hammersmith Hospital IVF Unit

Professor of Fertility Studies at Imperial College, he is also Director of NHS Research & Development for Hammersmith Hospital. Part of the first 'test-tube baby' team in '78, he performed the first successful experimental ovarian and tubal transplant and human tubal transplant, and helped develop gynaecological microsurgery. His group's research resulted in the first births after DNA testing to avoid sex-linked disease and single gene defects, and after PGD for chromosome defects. His team is developing methods for maturing eggs outside the body to make IVF cheaper and less intrusive.

Mr Patrick Steptoe and Professor Robert Edwards

Professor Edwards and the late Mr Steptoe, both gynaecologists, developed IVF to produce the world's first 'test-tube baby', Louise Brown, in '78. Mr Steptoe helped develop laparoscopy which he used for egg collection. Professor Edwards began researching fertility in '55, discovering how to manipulate hormone cycles and ways in which fertilisation and early embryo growth could occur outside the body. His experiments helped establish the timing of important stages in fertilisation and pregnancy. Together they manipulated hormone levels controlling the menstrual cycle, obtained mature eggs by laparoscopy, identified the proper time to fertilise them in a culture dish, developed the embryos in the laboratory and transferred them, with eventual success in '78. They founded Bourn Hall Clinic in 1980.

Regional index of clinics

South East

Canterbury, BMI Chaucer Hospital 185
Croydon, BMI Shirley Oaks Hospital 189
Eastbourne, Esperance Private Hospital 205
Great Missenden, BMI Chiltern Hospital 187
Orpington, BMI Chelsfield Park Hospital 186
Oxford, Oxford Fertility Unit 229
Sidcup, Queen Mary's Hospital 233
Southampton, Wessex Fertility Services/BUPA Chalybeate IVF Unit 246
West Malling, Maidstone Fertility Centre 222
Wexham, Thames Valley Nuffield Hospital 240
Woking, Woking Nuffield Hospital 250

South West

Bath, Bath Assisted Conception Clinic 181
Bristol, Bristol University 193
Bristol, Southmead Hospital 235
Bristol, Tower House Clinic 241
Dorchester, Winterbourne Fertility Centre 248
Exeter, Peninsular Centre for Reproductive Medicine 230
Plymouth, South West Centre for Reproductive Medicine 236

Trent

Leicester, Middle England Fertility Centre 224
Nottingham, CARE at the Park Hospital 196
Nottingham, NURTURE 228
Northampton, CARE at the Three Shires 197
Sheffield, Centre for Reproductive Medicine & Fertility 199

West Midlands

Aldridge, Midland Fertility Services 225
Birmingham, Birmingham Women's Hospital 183
Birmingham, BMI Priory Hospital 188
Bishop Auckland, Bishop Auckland Fertility Centre 184
Burton upon Trent, Burton Centre for Reproductive Medicine 194
Coventry, Centre for Reproductive Medicine 198
Hartlepool, Hartlepool General Hospital 209
Middlesborough, James Cook University Hospital 213
Newcastle under Lyme, North Staffordshire Nuffield Hospital 227
Shrewsbury, Shropshire & Mid-Wales Fertility Centre 234
Stokesley, Cleveland Gynaecology & Fertility Centre 201
Sunderland, Sunderland Fertility Centre 239
Wolverhampton, St Jude's Clinic for Fertility & Gynaecology 238
Wolverhampton, Wolverhampton Assisted Conception Unit 252

Wales

Bridgend, Princess of Wales Hospital 255
Cardiff, Cardiff Assisted Reproduction Unit 253
Swansea, Cromwell IVF & Fertility Centre 254

Scotland

Aberdeen, University of Aberdeen 258
Dundee, Ninewells Hospital 257
Glasgow, Glasgow Royal Infirmary 256

Useful addresses

ACeBabes
www.acebabes.co.uk
Helene Torr
31 Hillview Road, Carlton
Nottingham NG4 1JX
Tel 0115 9879266
Doriver Lilley
8 Yarwell Close, Derwent Heights
Derby DE21 4SW
Tel 01332 832558

ARC (formerly SATFA)
Antenatal Results & Choices
73 Charlotte Street
London W1T 4PN.
Helpline 020 7631 0285
www.arc-uk.org/

BAAF
**British Association for Adoption
and Fostering**
Skyline House, 200 Union Street
London SE1 0LX
Tel 020 7593 2000
www.baaf.org.uk

BICA
**British Infertility Counselling
Association**
69 Division Street
Sheffield S1 4GE
Tel 01342 843880
www.bica.net
info@bica.net

CHILD
**The National Infertility Support
Network**
Charter House, St Leonards Road
Bexhill on Sea, East Sussex TN40 1JA
Tel 01424 732361
www.child.org.uk
Email: office@child.org.uk

COTS
**Childlessness Overcome Through
Surrogacy**
Lairg
Sutherland IV27 4EF
Tel 0870 845 9048
www.surrogacy.org.uk
Email: info@surrogacy.org.uk

The Daisy Network
**For women suffering premature
menopause**
c/o CARE at the Park Hospital
Sherwood Lodge Drive
Burntstump Country Park, Arnold
Nottingham NG5 8RX
www.daisynetwork.org.uk
Email: info@daisynetwork.org.uk

Donor Conception Network
PO Box 265
Sheffield S3 7YX
Tel 020 8245 4369
www.dcnetwork.org

**The Electronic Infertility
Network**
Woodlawn House, Carrickfergus
Co. Antrim, Northern Ireland BT3 8PX
Tel 07885 138101
www.ein.org
Email: webmaster@ein.org

The Fostering Network
87 Blackfriars Road
London SE1 8HA
Tel: 020 7620 6400
www.thefostering.net
Email: penny.king@fostering.net

**The Fostering Network in
Scotland**
Ingram House, 2nd floor
227 Ingram Street, Glasgow
Scotland G1 1DA
Tel 0141 204 1400

**The Fostering Network in
Northern Ireland**
216 Belmont Road, Belfast
Northern Ireland BT4 2AT
Tel 028 9067 3441

HFEA
**Human Fertilisation and Embryology
Authority**
Paxton House
30 Artillery Lane
London E1 7LS
Tel 020 7377 5077
www.hfea.gov.uk
Email: admin@hfea.gov.uk

ISSUE
The National Fertility Association
114 Lichfield Street, Walsall
West Midlands WS1 1SZ
Tel 01922 722 888
www.issue.co.uk

The Miscarriage Association
c/o Clayton Hospital, Northgate
Wakefield, West Yorkshire WF1 3JS
Helpline 01924 200799
www.miscarriageassociation.org.uk
Email:
miscarriageassociation@care4free.net

MoreToLife
Support for the involuntarily childless
114 Lichfield Street
Walsall, WS1 1SZ
Tel 01922 722 888
www.moretolife.co.uk
Email: Diane@moretolife.co.uk

The National Endometriosis Society
Suite 50, Westminster Palace Gardens
1-7 Artillery Row, London SW1P 1RL
Freephone helpline 0808 808 2227
www.endo.org.uk

NGDT
The National Gamete Donation Trust
PO Box 137
Manchester M13 0YX
Tel 0161 276 6000
www.ngdt.inuk.com
Email: ngdtenq@aol.com

NIAC
National Infertility Awareness Campaign
www.ein.org/niac.htm

TAMBA
Twins And Multiple Births Association
2 The Willows, Gardner Road
Guildford, Surrey GU1 4PG
Tel 0870 770 3305
www.tamba.org.uk
Email: enquiries@tamba.org

Verity
The Polycystic Ovaries Self-Help Group
52-54 Featherstone Street
London EC1Y 8RT
www.verity-pcos.org.uk

**British Homeopathic Association
& the Faculty of Homeopathy**
Faculty members are medically trained
healthcare professionals such as GPs
Tel 020 7566 7800 (BHA)/7810 (Faculty)
www.trusthomeopathy.org

Society of Homeopaths
Society members have completed
homeopathic degree but may have no
other healthcare training
Tel 01604 621400
www.homeopathy-soh.org

The British Acupuncture Council
Members have over 1200 hours of
training and abide by a code of practice
Tel 020 8735 0400
www.acupuncture.org.uk

British Medical Acupuncture Society
Members practise acupuncture within
the scope of their medical training
Tel 01925 730727
www.medical-acupuncture.co.uk

The Acupuncture Association of Chartered Physiotherapists
Members practise acupuncture within
the scope of their medical training
Tel 01747 861151
www.aacp.uk.com

British Hypnotherapy Association
Sets standards in training and practice
Tel 020 7723 4443

The Register of Chinese Herbal Medicine
Members are qualified in Chinese medicine after studying for up to four years
Tel 01603 623994
www.rchm.co.uk

**Members of these Western herbal-
ist professional bodies are trained
to a minimum of degree level:**

The National Institute of Medical Herbalists
Tel 01392 426022
www.nimh.org.uk

Association of Master Herbalists
Tel 01482 887352

The International Register of Consultant Herbalists
Tel 01792 655886
www.irch.org

Glossary

Anovulation Failure to ovulate caused by medical conditions such as polycystic ovary syndrome or premature menopause.

Antibodies Proteins made by the body to fight or attack foreign substances entering the body. Normally they prevent infection; however, they can attack sperm or embryos.

Antiphospholipid antibodies Antibodies which attack phospholipids. In pregnancy, phospholipids act like a sort of glue that holds the dividing cells together, and are necessary for growth of the placenta into the wall of the uterus. Phospholipids also filter nourishment from the mother's blood to the baby, and filter the baby's waste back through the placenta. The antibodies themselves do not cause miscarriage, but their presence indicates that an abnormal autoimmune process may interrupt the ability of the phospholipids to do their job, putting the woman at risk of miscarriage, second trimester loss, intrauterine growth retardation (IUGR) and pre-eclampsia. They can be identified by blood tests.

Anti-sperm antibodies These attach themselves to sperm and inhibit their movement and ability to fertilise. Either the man or the woman may produce sperm antibodies. They are detected by an **Immunobead Binding Test (IBD)**.

Assisted conception Medical intervention to help achieve a pregnancy. Fertility treatment techniques such as in vitro fertilisation (IVF), IUI, GIFT, ZIFT and MAF may be used. Also called Assisted Reproduction (AR) or Assisted Reproductive Technology (ART).

Assisted hatching A small hole in the shell (zona pellucida) of the egg is created in vitro (outside the body). It aims to help the embryo hatch out of its shell and increase the chance of implantation. Often used in older women where the eggs may have tougher shells.

Azoospermia Complete absence of sperm in semen.

Basal body temperature (BBT) Your body temperature when taken at its lowest point, usually in the morning before getting out of bed. Charting BBT is used to predict ovulation.

Blastocyst An embryo that has developed for five days after fertilisation. The surface cells will become the placenta and the inner cell mass will become the fetus. A healthy blastocyst should hatch from the zona pellucida by the end of the sixth day. Within about 24 hours of hatching, it should begin to implant into the lining of the uterus.

Blastocyst transfer Allowing in vitro fertilised embryos to reach blastocyst stage (see above), usually five days, before transferring them into the uterus.

Buserelin A hormone suppressant given by nasal spray or a daily injection. It suppresses the activity of the pituitary gland which normally stimulates the ovaries to produce eggs. The ovaries can then be stimulated artificially.

Cervical mucus Secretions produced by the cells of the cervix around the cervical canal. Amount and texture change during ovulation to help sperm movement and fertilisation.

Cervix The opening between the uterus and the vagina. It acts as a reservoir for sperm and secretes an alkaline mucus to protect them from the acidic conditions of the vagina. It remains closed during pregnancy and dilates during labour to allow the baby to be born.

Chemical pregnancy A pregnancy whereby HCG levels are detected but the pregnancy is lost before a fetal heartbeat is seen on an ultrasound. This is a very early miscarriage, often occurring before the woman misses a period.

Chlamydia A sexually transmitted disease, it is a common cause of pelvic infection and subsequent tubal damage and infertility.

Chocolate cyst A cyst in the ovary that is filled with old blood. Also called an endometrioma. It occurs when endometriosis invades an ovary, causing it to swell. Often patients with endometriomas will not have any symptoms. If the cyst ruptures or the ovary containing it twists, however, emergency surgery may be required.

Chromosomes Tiny structures within cells that contain the genetic material that controls all the functions and characteristics of that particular cell. Sperm and egg cells contain 23 chromosomes each (half the number of normal body cells). When a sperm fertilises an egg, they combine to create a cell with the normal number of chromosomes, half from each parent.

Chromosome analysis Also known as karyotyping. Cells from parental eggs and sperm or from a fetus are studied to find abnormalities in the chromosomes that might be the underlying cause of repeated pregnancy losses.

Clinical pregnancy Detection of a fetal heartbeat using ultrasound.

Clomiphene (Clomid) Commonly used anti-estrogen drug, administered orally, which induces ovulation.

CMV – cytomegalovirus A group of viruses that cause enlargement of the cells of various organs. The virus, one of the herpes family, is extremely common. The infection can cause an illness similar to glandular fever, although in most cases there are no symptoms. A pregnant woman who contracts the disease can pass the virus on to the unborn baby and in rare cases this can cause malformations and brain damage.

Conception The fertilisation of an egg by a sperm, forming an embryo or zygote.

Controlled Ovarian Hyperstimulation Use of fertility drugs to stimulate the growth of multiple follicles for ovulation. Also called superovualtion.

Corpus luteum The yellow-coloured glandular structure that forms from the ovarian follicle after ovulation. It produces the hormone progesterone, so if the corpus luteum is functioning poorly and there is a deficiency in the amount of progesterone produced, or the length of time it is produced for, the endometrium may not be able to support a pregnancy.

Cryopreservation The freezing of oocytes, spermatozoa or embryos and their storage in liquid nitrogen.

Cystic fibrosis An inherited genetic disorder that affects a number of organs in the body (especially the lungs and pancreas) by clogging them with thick, sticky mucus.

D&C (dilatation and curettage) A procedure in which the cervical canal is expanded (dilated) and the lining and the contents of the womb are scraped out. This may be done to diagnose or treat abnormal bleeding and to help prevent infection. It is usually performed under a general anaesthetic.

DI – Donor Insemination The insertion of donated sperm into the vagina, cervix or womb. Used if the male partner has few or no sperm, or risks passing on an inherited disease.

Dummy cycle A 'practice' treatment cycle. It may be done in a natural ovulatory cycle or in a cycle modified by a combination of hormone tablets and injections. It ensures that the uterus can be adequately primed to achieve successful implantation.

Ectopic pregnancy Abnormal pregnancy in which a fertilised egg implants outside the uterus – usually in one of the fallopian tubes, the ovary or the abdominal cavity.

Egg collection Procedure in which eggs are taken from a woman's ovaries using an ultrasound-guided needle or a laparoscope and a needle. Also known as egg retrieval.

Embryo A fertilised egg of up to eight weeks development.

Embryo biopsy Removal and examination of one or more cells from a developing embryo for diagnostic purposes.

Embryo donation This may be offered when there are male and/or female problems, or there is a high risk of passing on a genetic disorder, making it difficult or impossible to have a child of their own. Embryos are donated by couples who have been undergoing assisted conception and wish to make any frozen embryos 'left over' available to other couples.

Embryo freezing Embryos not required for treatment in a cycle can be frozen in liquid nitrogen and stored for future use. Also known as **cryopreservation** or embryo storage.

Embryo grading Fertilised eggs are examined by an embryologist to assess their development. Embryos with the highest score have round, symmetrical cells, and give high pregnancy rates when transferred back to the uterus.

Infertility Defined as the inability to conceive after a year of intercourse without contraception for a woman under 35, or after six months for women over 35, or the inability to carry a pregnancy to term.

Intramuscular injection An injection into a muscle (as opposed to into the skin or vein).

IUI intra-uterine insemination. Involves placing a sample of prepared sperm in the uterus via the cervix (neck of the womb), thereby bypassing cervical mucus (which may be hostile) and overcoming sperm count and/or motility problems.

IVF in vitro fertilisation. Eggs and sperm are collected and mixed together to achieve fertilisation outside the body. Sometimes known as the 'test-tube technique', although fertilisation actually takes place in a glass petri dish rather than a test tube.

IVF cycle Follows the same period of time as a menstrual cycle, but the processes are enhanced, maximising the potential for fertilisation. This involves the careful stimulation of various hormones at specific times during the 28 days. As in the menstrual cycle, the cycle is over if there is a menstrual period at the end of the 28 days rather than a pregnancy.

Kallman's Syndrome A congenital dysfunction of the hypothalamus with symptoms including failure to complete puberty.

Klinefelter's Syndrome A genetic abnormality wherein a carrier has one Y (male) chromosome and two X (female) chromosomes or a combination of 46XY and 47 XX chromosomes (a mosaic). It often causes fertility problems and can be passed on genetically.

Laparoscope A slender telescopic device that is inserted through an incision in the abdominal wall to view the abdominal or pelvic cavities. Used to diagnose a number of problems affecting fertility ie endometriosis and polycystic ovaries, and in egg retrieval.

Laparoscopic ovarian diathermy (LOD) A surgical treatment for PCOS, offered to women with clomiphene-resistant PCOS. It involves applying a short burst of diathermy (heat) or laser treatment to the surface of each ovary at multiple points. The hormone changes that this induces encourage the ovaries to ovulate spontaneously.

Laparoscopy A surgical procedure using a laparoscope (see above) inserted through a small incision in the abdominal wall. This is usually performed under a general anaesthetic.

Live birth rate The number of live births achieved from every 100 treatment cycles commenced. The Adjusted Live Birth Rate is the number of live births per 100 treatment cycles after adjustment to allow for the different types of patient treated eg different ages.

Luteal phase The post-ovulatory phase of a woman's menstrual cycle. The corpus luteum produces progesterone which causes the thickening of the uterine lining in readiness to support the implantation and growth of an embryo.

Luteal phase defect Occurs when the uterine lining does not develop adequately, due either to inadequate progesterone stimulation or because the uterine lining is unable to respond to progesterone. It may prevent embryo implantation or cause early miscarriage.

Luteinising hormone (LH) Stimulates ovulation in women and the production of the sex hormone testosterone in men.

Menopause The transition period in a woman's life when the ovaries stop producing eggs, menstrual activity decreases and eventually ceases, and the body decreases the production of the hormones oestrogen and progesterone.

Menstrual cycle A cycle occurring over a period of approximately one month during which an egg is released from an ovary and the uterus prepares to receive a fertilised egg. The blood and tissue of the uterus lining are lost through the vagina if pregnancy does not occur.

MESA - Micro Epididymal Sperm Aspiration Retrieval of sperm from the epididymis by making a small incision in the scrotum and extracting fluid from the epididymis

Micro-Assisted Fertilisation (MAF) This term refers to any technique used in IVF to bypass the zona pellucida of the egg. ICSI is the most commonly used MAF technique but others such as SUZI are also used. Such techniques are also known as micromanipulation.

Microsurgical Epididymal Sperm Aspiration (MESA) see MESA and **Sperm retrieval**.

Miscarriage Spontaneous total loss of a pregnancy before 24 weeks of gestation.

Mittelschmerz Pain or discomfort on one or both sides of the abdomen at ovulation.

Motility A measure of how active sperm are.

Multiple birth rate The percentage of all births in which more than one baby was born.

Multiple pregnancy rate Calculated as a proportion of all clinical pregnancies.

Mutation A change or changes in a gene or chromosome that cause a disorder or an inherited susceptibility to a disorder.

Natural cycle IVF Collecting and fertilising an egg ovulated during a natural menstrual cycle.

Non-surgical sperm aspiration (NSA) A small needle is used to extract sperm directly from the testis. Used in IVF and ICSI for men who cannot ejaculate or have blocked ducts.

Obstetrician-Gynaecologist A doctor specialising in the diseases and routine physical care of the female reproductive system including treatment through pregnancy and childbirth.

Oestrogen Female sex hormone formed in the ovary, responsible for the development of female secondary sex characteristics. During the menstrual cycle it works to produce suitable conditions for the fertilisation, implantation and nutrition of an embryo.

Oligomenorrhea Infrequent menstrual periods

Oligo-ovulation Infrequent ovulation (usually fewer than 6 times per year).

Oligospermia Having few sperm.

Oocyte The female egg or reproductive cell, also known as the **ovum.**

Oophorectomy Surgical removal of the ovaries.

Ovarian cyst A very common condition in which fluid collects in a sac in the ovary.

Ovarian cyst aspiration An ultrasound-guided needle is introduced into the cyst through the vagina. The fluid contents of the cyst are then drawn out of the ovary through the needle.

Ovarian drilling Used to treat androgen levels and restore cycles in women with polycystic ovaries. An electrosurgery needle burns small holes into the ovaries during a laparoscopy.

Ovarian failure Diagnosed by elevated FSH levels in the blood, it is the failure of the ovary to respond to FSH stimulation from the pituitary, due to damage or malformation of the ovary.

Ovarian hyperstimulation syndrome (OHSS) Some women may over-respond to the drugs given to them to stimulate ovulation. This can cause abdominal pain/swelling and occasionally cysts on the ovaries. In rare severe cases, large numbers of eggs develop and the ovaries swell. In these circumstances, hospital admission would be required.

Ovulation The release of an egg from the ovaries.

Ovulation induction Treatment, usually with drugs, to stimulate ovulation, particularly if a woman is not producing eggs regularly.

Partial Zonal Dissection (PZD) A type of IVF treatment in which a hole is made in the outer shell of the egg with a glass needle, helping the sperm to penetrate the egg.

Pelvic Inflammatory Disease (PID) An infection of the pelvic organs causing high fever and extreme pain and illness. PID can lead to tubal blockage and pelvic adhesions.

Pelvic ultrasound scan An ultrasound performed by moving the transducer across the abdomen (transabdominal scan). The transducer can also be placed in a man's rectum (transrectal scan) or in a woman's vagina (transvaginal scan).

Perimenopause The two to 15 years before menopause during which a woman experiences changes due to declining levels of oestrogen and progesterone.

Persona system Persona is actually intended as a way to help you avoid conception. It works by measuring levels of FSH and LH in order to predict when conception is likely so that couples can have sex without using protection at other times of the month. Therefore it can also help to predict when you are ovulating and at your most fertile.

PESA - Percutaneous Epididymal Sperm Aspiration A form of sperm retrieval where a small needle is passed directly into the epididymis under local anaesthetic and fluid is drawn out. If the fluid contains any sperm these are used for ICSI (see **Sperm retrieval**).

Pituitary gland The gland that stimulates the action of all other glands in the body.

Placenta Embryonic tissue that implants in the uterine wall. The fetus is attached to the placenta via the umbilical cord, providing the mechanism for exchanging the waste product (including carbon dioxide) of the baby for the nutrients and oxygen of the mother.

Polycystic ovary syndrome (PCOS) PCOS happens when the ovaries have many small follicles containing eggs that have stopped growing. Symptoms may include excessive weight, acne and increased body hair or hair thinning. It results in high LH levels, low FSH levels and higher than usual production of androgen hormones. Because ovulation is not happening, progesterone is no longer produced, although oestrogen levels remain normal.

Post-coital test Also known as the cervical mucus sperm penetration test, it is carried out on the woman and determines the sperm's ability to swim through the mucus in the cervix.

Premature ovarian failure (POF) A loss of ovarian function in women under 40. Periods stop, oestrogen is low and the follicle-stimulating hormone (FSH) level is elevated.

Prenatal testing Tests used to check the health of the developing fetus and to test for any genetic abnormalities. These include: amniocentesis, nuchal scanning and blood testing. These can be done at different stages in the development of the fetus.

Primary Care Trust (PCT) These are responsible for the planning and securing of health services and improving the health of the local population. For example, PCTs must make sure there are enough GPs to provide for their population and that they are accessible to patients. They are responsible for integrating health and social care so the two systems work together for patients. The PCTs in England will be given funding to plan and commission local health services – a role previously carried out by health authorities.

Primary infertility Inability to conceive at all, affects between two–10 per cent of couples.

Progesterone Female sex hormone produced during the second half of the menstrual cycle. It is responsible for preparing and supporting the uterine lining for implantation.

Prostate gland A gland (approx. 3.5-4.0 cm) found in males. It surrounds the neck of the bladder and the urethra. The prostate gland secretes a third of the fluid that makes up semen.

Resistant Ovary Syndrome A condition in which the ovary is unable to respond to the stimulus sent out by FSH to its follicle.

Retroverted uterus The uterus is tipped backwards towards the rectum.

Salpingectomy Surgical removal of the fallopian tubes.

Salpingography A test used to assess the outline of the uterus and check whether the fallopian tubes are open. The procedure usually involves passing catheters into each fallopian tube. An X-ray machine then images the catheters, and dye is injected into each fallopian tube. The dye is observed as it passes through the fallopian tube and hopefully out into the abdominal cavity. If this occurs, then the fallopian tube is open.

Salpingitis Inflammation of one or both fallopian tubes.

Salpingolysis Surgery to remove adhesions restricting the movement and functions of reproductive organs.

Saline examination of uterine cavity Hysterosonography/sonohystogram (saline infusion sonography) is a relatively new procedure in which sterile saline is injected into the uterus while a transvaginal sonograph is performed. The purpose is to distend the uterine cavity (endometrial cavity) to look for polyps, fibroids or cancer, especially in patients with abnormal uterine bleeding. Another version of this procedure uses saline solution and air. These are injected into the uterus and the physician looks for air bubbles passing through the fallopian tubes, which shows whether or not the fallopian tubes are open.

Satellite IVF If you live far from the clinic, ovulation stimulation can be monitored by one nearer home. Egg collection may take place in either, embryo transfer always takes place at the IVF clinic.

Secondary infertility The inability to conceive or maintain a pregnancy after previously having had one or more children. The term is also applied to women who have had one or more miscarriages or stillbirths. Secondary infertility is more common than primary infertility. It is estimated that 10 to 25 per cent of couples have secondary infertility.

Semen analysis A laboratory test done to assess the quality of semen. The quantity, concentration, form and motility of sperm will be tested. The volume of semen will also be measured and checked for white blood cells, which may indicate an infection.

Semen (seminal fluid) Fluid released by the male at orgasm containing sperm and secretions from the prostate gland.

Seminal vesicles A pair of glands at the base of the bladder that secrete seminal fluid and nourish and promote the movement of sperm through the urethra.

Seminiferous tubules A network of tubules in the testicles in which sperm are made, mature and move towards the epididymis for storage until their release.

Sonogram Also known as ultrasound. This is the use of high-frequency sound waves to create an image of internal body parts. Can detect follicle growth and monitor pregnancy.

Sperm Male reproductive cell that carries genetic information to the female egg.

Spermatid An immature sperm.

Sperm bank Place where sperm are stored frozen in liquid nitrogen for later use.

Sperm count Number of sperm in semen, sometimes known as sperm concentration or sperm density. The number is given as the number of sperm per millilitre.

Sperm invasion test A sample of semen and cervical mucus are placed next to each other on a glass slide and this is observed under a microscope. If the mucus is hostile to the sperm, the sperm may have difficulty swimming into the mucus and any that do may stop moving.

Sperm morphology One of the factors measured in a sperm analysis, it is a calculation of how many or what percentage of sperm in a sample appear to have been formed normally.

Sperm motility The ability of sperm to swim.

Sperm penetration The ability of sperm to penetrate the zona pellucida of the egg.

Sperm retrieval (PESA, MESA, TESE or FROSTESE) If there is no sperm present in the semen (because of obstruction or other forms of azoospermia), it is sometimes possible to collect sperm from inside the reproductive organs, by using **PESA, MESA, TESE** or **FROSTESE**.

Sperm washing Separating sperm from semen and motile from non-motile sperm.

Subfertility Very few couples are truly infertile. Most of those who seek help are actually subfertile – that is they have problems that make it unlikely they will conceive without medical help. The term also includes women who are able to conceive but have trouble carrying a baby to term because of recurrent miscarriage.

Superovulation Fertility drugs stimulate the ovaries into producing more mature eggs than the one they would normally. Also known as **Controlled Ovarian Hyperstimulation**.

Surrogacy A surrogate ('host') mother is inseminated with the sperm of the intended father either by means of artificial insemination or (more rarely) by having sex with the male partner. The host mother is the genetic mother of the child, while the intended father is the genetic father. A variation is to use donated sperm or the 'host' mother carries a baby after IVF or GIFT using sperm and eggs from the intended parents of the child. The child is the genetic child of the commissioning couple and has no genetic relationship to the 'host' mother. There is yet another option which is gestational surrogacy using a donor egg whereby the embryo is created from a donor egg and the sperm of the intended father.

SUZI - Sub-Zonal Insemination A forerunner of ICSI whereby sperm is injected underneath the egg's zona pellucida.

Testes The male reproductive organs which produce sperm. They are also endocrine glands.

Testicle The male gonad, producing sperm and the hormone testosterone.

Testicular biopsy A minor surgical procedure in which a small sample of testicular tissue is taken for examination. Carries a possibility of damage to the testes.

Testicular enzyme defect Congenital defect which prevents the testes responding to hormonal stimulation, resulting in oligospermia or azoospermia.

Testicular failure Primary failure is congenital, developmental or stemming from a genetic error causing a malformation that prevents sperm production. Secondary failure is a result of acquired testicular damage, for example from drugs or exposure to toxic substances or physical damage such as varicocoele.

TESE - Testicular Sperm Extraction A form of sperm retrieval whereby a biopsy is done on the testicle to find sperm cells.

Testosterone A male sex hormone produced by the testes that is responsible for the sex drive, and also causes male sexual characteristics such as hair growth, muscles and deep voice.

Total effective sperm count Estimate of the number of sperm capable of fertilization.

Trial embryo transfer A catheter is passed through the cervix into the uterus to determine its path through the cervix and to measure the distance to the top of the uterine cavity. It will also help determine any likely problems so these can be avoided during the real thing.

Tubal patency Open, unobstructed fallopian tubes.

Tuboplasty Reconstructive or plastic surgery to correct abnormalities of the fallopian tubes which may be causing blockage or otherwise affecting fertility.

Turner's Syndrome The most common cause of genetic female fertility problems. The woman will have only one X chromosome or a mosaic (46XX and 45X). As a result the ovaries will fail to form, instead appearing as thin threads of deteriorated ovarian tissue.

Ultrasound scan See also **Sonogram**.

Undescended testes When the testicles have failed to descend from the abdominal cavity into the scrotum by the age of one. If not repaired, this may result in permanent infertility.

Unexplained fertility See **Idiopathic fertility**.

Urethra Tube through which urine passes between the bladder and the outside of the body. In men this tube also carries semen.

Urologist Doctor specialising in the urinary system and male reproductive system.

Uterus Also known as the womb, this is the hollow muscular female reproductive organ which houses and nourishes a fetus during pregnancy.

Varicocele Dilatation and swelling of the veins which drain the testicle and may cause a bulge above the testicle in the scrotum or aching and discomfort. It usually affects the left testis and can result in high temperature in the testis as a result of blood pooling in the tests. This in turn can lead to a low sperm count.

Vas deferens The tubes along which sperm pass from the testes to the epididymis.

Vasectomy Removal of all or part of the vas deferens, usually as a means of sterilisation.

Vasectomy reversal Surgical repair of the vas deferens to restore fertility.

Viral screen Blood tests to check for various viruses that can affect fertility or the health of a potential fetus (for example, hepatitis B & C, HIV, rubella, VDRL).

X chromosome The genetic matter in a cell that provides the necessary information to make a female. All eggs contain one X chromosome and half of all sperm carry an X chromosome. When two X chromosomes combine, the resultant fetus will be female.

X-linked disorders Disorders that occur due to a mutation on the X chromosome. These only usually affect males, but they can be transmitted through a healthy female 'carrier'.

Y chromosome The genetic matter in a cell that provides the necessary information to make a male. The Y chromosome is found in half of a man's sperm cells, so if one of these combine with the X chromosome of the egg, a male (XY) fetus will be produced.

ZIFT - Zygote Intrafallopain Transfer An assisted conception technique where fertilisation takes place in the laboratory (as with IVF). However, the fertilised eggs are transferred directly into the fallopain tubes on day one after fertilisation, the idea being that this is where the embryo would be developing in a natural pregnancy.

Zona pellucida The protective membrane or 'shell' surrounding the egg.

Zygote Medical term for an egg that has fertilised but not yet divided.

INDEX

HIV 42, 131
HMG (human menopausal gonadotrophin) 71-2
Hormones 9-12, 118
  blood tests 48-9
HSG (hysterosalpingogram) 46, 47, 49
Humegon see HMG (human menopausal gonadotrophin)
HyCoSy (hysterosalpingo-contrast sonography) 51-2
Hydrosalpinx 63
Hyperprolactinaemia 58, 69
Hypnotherapy 61, 66, 87
Hypogonadotrophic hypogonadism 68-9
Hypopituitarism 68
Hypothalamus 10, 12
Hypothyroidism see Thyroid problems
Hysterectomy 138
Hysterosalpingogram see HSG
Hysteroscopy 46, 50, 59
ICSH (interstitial cell-stimulating hormone) 12
ICSI (intracytoplasmic sperm injection) 55, 65, 81, 86-7, 93, 104-5
Idiopathic (unexplained) fertility 4, 65-6, 88, 90, 103, 128
Immune system 13
  abnormalities 118, 119
Implantation 4, 11-12
In vitro fertilisation see IVF
Infertility
  causes 18
  coping with 148-57
  definition 18
  primary 19, 90
  rate 2-3, 19-20
  secondary 19, 90
Inflammatory bowel disease 22, 23
Inhibin 12
Insemination
  artificial 89
  donor 81
  interuterine see IUI
  intracervical 89
  sub-zonal 81, 105
Internet 115
Interstitial cells 12
Interuterine insemination see IUI
Intracervical insemination 89
ISSUE 6, 107, 149, 157, 266
IUI (interuterine insemination) 58, 81, 83, 88-9, 128, 161
IUI-D (IUI with donor) 81
IVF (in vitro fertilisation) 3, 58, 81, 82, 86-7, 89-99
  assisted hatching 98
  blastocyst transfer 96-7
  cancellation of treatment 99
  cost 5, 100, 145, 163
  donor assisted conception 123
  egg-sharing 5, 166
  fallopian tubes, removal 63-4
  and fertility drugs 91
  labelling and checking procedures 97
  miscarriage rate 4, 113, 116
  multiple pregnancy 94-5
  natural cycle 99-100
  overseas treatment 94

  sex during treatment 95
  success rate 90-1
  surrogacy 139
  technique 92-8
  treatment failure 120-2
Keyhole surgery 59
Laparoscopic microsurgery 59
Laparoscopy and dye 46, 47, 50-1
Laparotomy 59
Legal position
  abroad 4-5, 41, 94, 131
  donor assisted conception 136
  surrogacy 138, 139-40
  in the UK 3, 67, 138
Lesbian couples 41, 42
Leuprolide acetate 79
LH (luteinising hormone) 10, 11, 12, 24, 71, 72, 74, 118, 119
  blood test 48
  drug treatment 70-1
Live birth rate 38
Low positive pregnancy test 108, 114
Luteal phase 59
  defect 59
Luteinising hormone see LH
MAF (micro-assisted fertilisation) 81, 104-5
Male fertility 12-13, 188
  and age 18, 21
  drug treatment 80
  medical problems affecting 22
Medical help, when to seek 26-27
Medication, effect on fertility 23
Menopause 11, 21
  perimenopause 21, 60-1
  premature see POF
  premenopausal symptoms 35
Menotrophins 78
Menstrual cycle 9-10, 11-12
  cervical mucus 24
  changes in 35
  length 30
  luteal phase 59
  mittelschmerz 25
  ovulation 9
  suppression by drugs 74, 92
Menstruation 12
  amenorrhoea 15, 22, 26, 58, 68
  dysmenorrhoea 15, 22
  irregular 15, 26, 35, 49, 58, 114, 152
MESA (micro epididymal sperm aspiration) 85
Metrodin see FSH (follicle-stimulation hormone)
Micro-assisted fertilisation see MAF
Microprolactinomas 58
Miscarriage 4, 15, 16, 19, 26, 59, 153
  following assisted conception 113-19
  missed 117
  rate 117
  recurrent 119, 124, 138
  threatened 115, 116
Mittelschmerz 25
MoreToLife 157, 266
Mucus, cervical see Cervical mucus
Multiple pregnancy 76, 84, 94-5, 111-13
  associated dangers 112
  rate 112